Get Gorgeous

21 DAYS TO A MORE BEAUTIFUL, CONFIDENT YOU

Design and Typesetting: Claude-Olivier Four
Translated from the French by Jeanne B. Cheynel

Editorial Directors: Kate Mascaro and Gaëlle Lassée
Editorial Assistance: Fanny Morgensztern,
Nadja Belhadj, Helen Adedotun
Color Separation: Bussière, Paris
Printed in China by Toppan Leefung

Simultaneously published in French
as *#Beauty Challenge: 21 jours pour être au top*
© Flammarion, S.A., Paris, 2016

English-language edition
© Flammarion, S.A., Paris, 2016

editions.flammarion.com

16 17 18   3 2 1

ISBN: 978-2-08-020265-9

Legal Deposit: 09/2016

CHRISTEL VATASSO
PASCAL LOPERENA

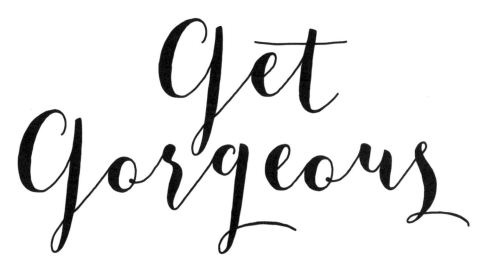

Get Gorgeous

21 DAYS TO A
MORE **BEAUTIFUL**,
CONFIDENT YOU

Flammarion

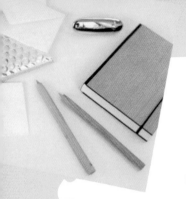

CONTENTS

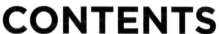

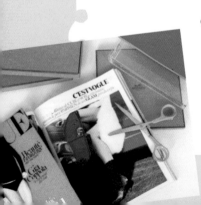

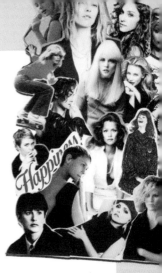
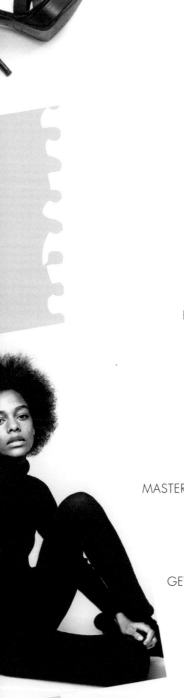

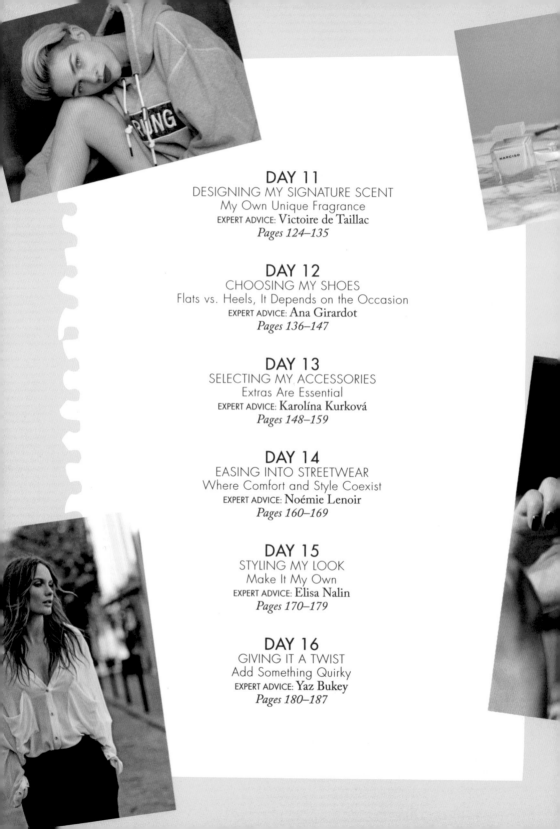

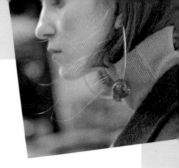

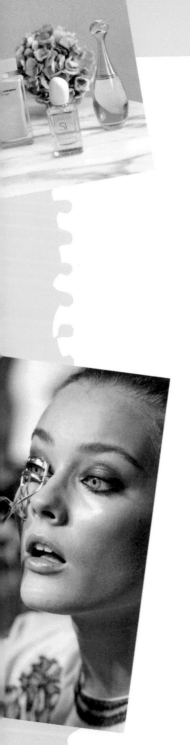

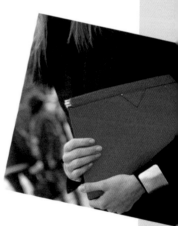

TWENTY-ONE DAYS TO GORGEOUS

I can't remember exactly what first sparked my quest for beauty—my fascination with beautiful objects and people and my preference for authentic feelings and emotions; simply put, my zest for life.

What is beauty? What are its main features? Does it lie in the eye of the beholder or can it be defined? Victor Hugo wrote: "Form is substance that rises to the surface." For me the search for beauty is not in the least bit superficial. Above all, it is a search for meaning through the aesthetics of form and feeling, a never-ending quest. "The eye has to travel," as Diana Vreeland says in her eponymous 2011 documentary film: be curious about everything, pay attention to others and to yourself, be inspired, have confidence in yourself, grow, be accomplished and fulfilled—isn't this what life is all about? We all know that perfection doesn't exist, but aiming for the best and following your dreams and desires are essential life goals. I see myself at age thirteen, leafing through magazines next to my mother and being struck by a photo of Eileen Ford, the modeling agency pioneer, surrounded by telephones. "Mom," I asked, "what's the job where you get to choose models?" What a surprise it was years later when I received a call from Ford Models in New York asking me to open the Paris branch of their agency. Surely this was destiny.

A few years ago Patrick Lemire, a well-known agent at Marilyn whose entire career was devoted to models, introduced me to Pascal Loperena. An artistic director and photographer, Pascal shared my passion for fashion, which naturally led to our collaboration at Ford. At the same time, my friend Gaëlle approached us with the idea of doing a modern take on a book like the one Eileen Ford published in the 1970s. Right away, Pascal and I were inspired by the idea of a book about fashion, beauty, and style.

We are aware that our industry can be the source of neuroses and complexes, so we wanted to speak out to encourage women to

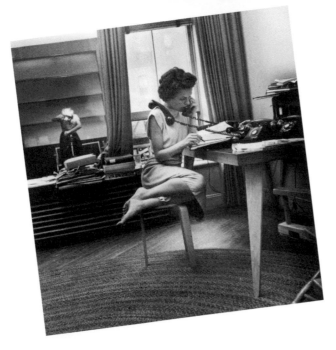

Eileen Ford in New York, 1948.

WHAT IS BEAUTY? WHAT ARE ITS MAIN FEATURES? DOES IT LIE IN THE EYE OF THE BEHOLDER OR CAN IT BE DEFINED?

find their own solutions to style and beauty questions. You don't have to follow fashion images to a T; everyone is free to find the style that suits them, without seeking perfection, but aiming for the best. It is not as unattainable as it seems to have an attractive body, great hair and skin, to feel gorgeous, smell good, own beautiful clothes, and live in charming surroundings.

Throughout our careers, our aim has been to search for the beauty around us and to enhance it. Seeing others at their best is a real pleasure, and because we are lucky enough to frequent the world's most gorgeous models, it's only natural that we wanted to create a guide to help all women find their bearings on the path to wellness and beauty. In this book, we combined our years of industry experience with that of the many wonderful people we've met in this incredible milieu in order to offer you our most precious recommendations.

A GUIDE TO MORE
SELF-KNOWLEDGE
AND SELF-LOVE

21 days to a more beautiful, confident you: this book is a guide to changing, evolving, finding yourself, and sharing with others. Why twenty-one days? Because the saying goes that it takes three weeks to change a habit. I've always been fascinated by the idea that we can change, and I've often observed that one thing holds true: everything is always possible.

Twenty-one days is also the amount of time we allot for a model to get prepared for a show: to learn to walk on three-inch heels, lose an inch or two around the waist, perk up a dull hairstyle, have a makeover, and get the hang of presenting herself. So we designed this book as a kind of daily challenge in calendar form, with each chapter corresponding to one day and one objective for the reader to tackle.

And because I was lucky enough all these years to encounter women who put love and passion into the world of fashion, I wanted to let them speak out, to get their expert opinions, but in a lighthearted way, using a Proustian questionnaire. I'm pleased to introduce you to these unique, inspiring women.

They may be fashion and beauty experts, but they are so much like us. They all agreed to take part and have shared their personal motto for living well.

Finally, we want you to use this book to track your wishes, ideas, and progress throughout this "wellness" pursuit. Being rather girly myself, I have always liked little notebooks and intimate diaries, which I use to jot down ideas and to glue in clippings of images, photos, and articles. That's why we designed the book as a sort of notebook for you—one that is yours and yours alone, that you can refer back to, daily. Like the children's books of your past, where you identified with the heroine, we want you to actively participate in this twenty-one day challenge, and to create a community of women brought together based on the theme of beauty. Throughout the book, you'll be invited to use the #getgorgeous and #beautychallenge21 hashtags when you post your daily progress and efforts on Instagram.

So let's get to it. Have fun. Set objectives, seek fulfillment, stop procrastinating, and venture into this beauty and wellness challenge.

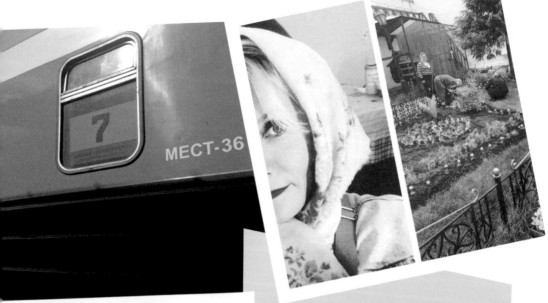

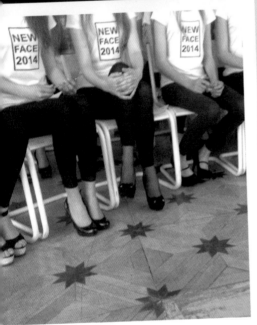

A NEW BEGINNING

I love traveling to scout for young women with modeling potential. Once, on a magical trip on the Trans-Siberian Railway to discover a future top model, I met an eighty year-old babushka who had been the guardian of the Krasnoyarsk chapel since her childhood. She told me her life story, all the while giving me good advice for my own life. A few hours later, I found myself standing in front of about one hundred girls from the surrounding villages, all impatiently awaiting my advice on how to become a model. Once the final cuts are made, and the selected girls arrive in Paris or New York, you would be surprised to see how rapidly they transform, as if by magic. And now you can, too!

DAY

01

GETTING

Started

MY PERSONAL ASSESSMENT

TAKE **STOCK**

"You'll never have a second chance
to make a good first impression."

David Swanson

A first impression. So often, we under-estimate this first (and last) chance to appear in our best light when we meet new people.

Yet that is the very thing an agent works on when we give a model a makeover. You'd be surprised to see how imperfect the women are at the start of the process. It's extremely rare for a young woman with no flaws to waltz into a modeling agency. Attaining perfection (if it exists!) is a difficult and ambitious goal, and whether it's even a desirable one is question-able. The path to achieving perfection often involves daily, regular teamwork between the model and her agents. I'm going to share all of my experience with you so that, together, we can bring out the best version of yourself.

I'm not suggesting that we should turn you into someone else; on the contrary, I want to see to it that you *tune in* to yourself.

In this first chapter, day one of the chal-lenge, you are going to take stock of who you are today, before you get started making any changes. You first have to take a good look at yourself, at your imperfections and weak-nesses. For starters, I'd like you to draw up an overall review of yourself, as you are today.

Jot down on paper—page 17 is just the place—the things you want to improve. Recording this precious information will help you keep track of how much ground you've covered and the progress you've made over the course of this challenge. Be honest with yourself from the start: there's no point in lying. If you're straightforward when con-fronting your flaws, you'll do a better job of correcting them.

Often modeling agencies are tempted to tell little lies—they erase a few centimeters from the size of one model's hips and add a bit to another's height. Cheating like this might initially feel good, but the punishment is terrible when the girls who don't meet the mark find themselves alongside those who fit the casting to a T.

Please understand: you are not judging yourself or dwelling on your flaws here, but getting to know yourself better. All the infor-mation you'll jot down in this notebook will remain OUR SECRET.

LET'S GO,
IT'S TIME TO GET
STARTED!

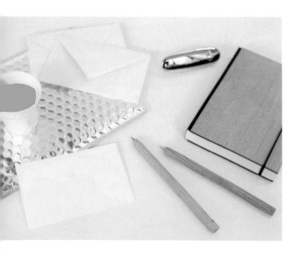

reveal your figure. Personally, I prefer taking photos to the torture of the tape measure any day! So grab your camera and take a:
- full-length photo of yourself;
- ¾ photo of your bust;
- portrait without makeup, your hair pulled back;
- portrait with your everyday makeup.

Or, you can employ a third personal assessment technique: identify your "reference" outfit: the one you wear when your weight is ideal, the one that makes you feel beautiful. The difference in just one buttonhole is enough to tell you when you've let yourself go!

I f you're feeling brave, you can do it like the pros and use a tape measure to take your measurements. Many models go pale at the sight of such things: it's a cruel, intimate moment, a reality check. Some of the models who come to us resist or even cry when we ask to take their measurements.

If the tape measure scares you, just take your picture in front of the mirror, instead. Our goal here is simple, really: all we want to do is keep a visual trace of where you stand on the first day of this challenge. For this exercise it's best to wear simple clothes: jeans and a white or black close-fitting top to

L ooking at yourself from head to toe is a first step. But to truly assess yourself, you have to get inside your head. What does it take to gain a sense of well-being? We only live once—unfortunately—and taking care of ourselves and those around us helps make life better. Happiness is not an end in itself, but a path, a road, a way to live. Visualizing yourself at your best, being demanding, having ambition, and seeking to evolve every day are a few keys to being beautiful.

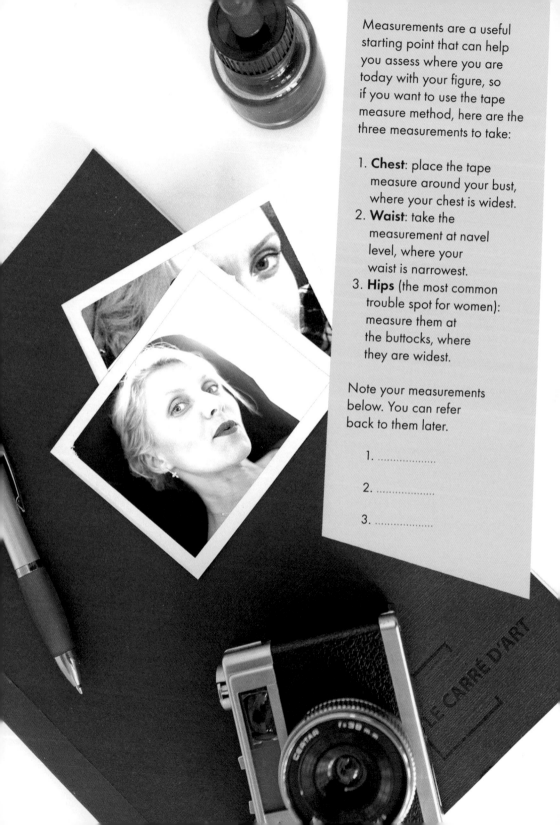

Measurements are a useful starting point that can help you assess where you are today with your figure, so if you want to use the tape measure method, here are the three measurements to take:

1. **Chest**: place the tape measure around your bust, where your chest is widest.
2. **Waist**: take the measurement at navel level, where your waist is narrowest.
3. **Hips** (the most common trouble spot for women): measure them at the buttocks, where they are widest.

Note your measurements below. You can refer back to them later.

1. ....

2. ....

3. ....

TAKE STOCK
OF YOUR **LIFE**

Now that you've reviewed where your body is today, here are a few recommendations for doing the same for your mind. How can you hope to feel beautiful if you're feeling down?

How old are you? What have you accomplished? What are your goals? Are you happy?

The point of this exercise is not to feel guilty but to reset the clocks. It's a good way to figure out where you stand. Write down your current situation and the one you are striving for. Identify your problems and hang-ups honestly: the aim is to draw positive conclusions in order to move forward. Free your mind: accepting its meanderings and desires is the first step toward wellness, self-esteem, and confidence.

Get rid of everything around you that you find displeasing. It's never too late to do the right thing! Identify the nuisances in your daily life, note them down, and change them. Clear your mind and pay attention to your real needs; hone in on your desires and free yourself of beliefs and attitudes that hamper your progress.

This challenge, I hope, will help you discover the diamond inside you so that, every day, you can shine a little more brightly. Like with photography, everything in life comes down to lighting and perspective!

So: in twenty-one days, are you ready to change for the rest of your life?

"IF YOU HAVE NOTHING AT ALL TO CREATE, THEN PERHAPS YOU CREATE YOURSELF."

CARL-GUSTAV JUNG

My Status

Today	In 21 Days
....	....
....	....
....	....
....	....
....	....
....	....
....	....
....	....
....	....
....	....
....	....
....	....
....	....

POST YOUR "BEFORE" PICTURE, SHOWING WHERE YOU ARE TODAY.
*#getgorgeous, #beautychallenge21*

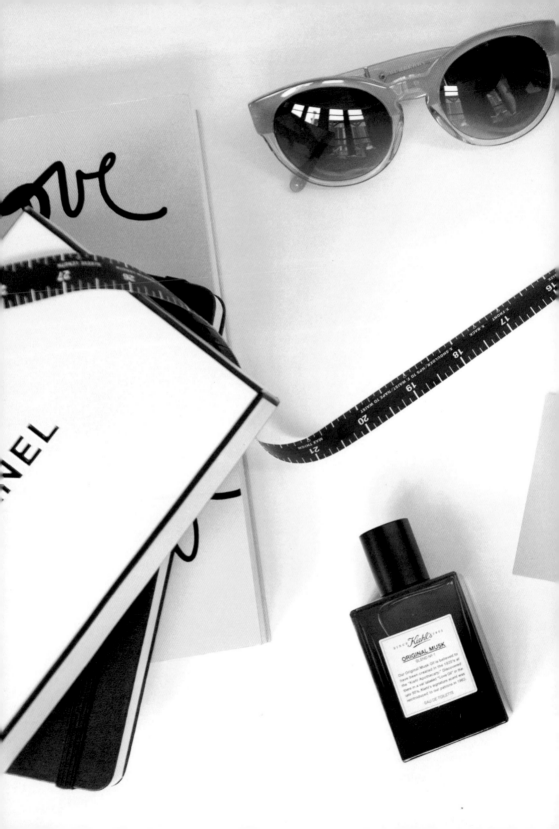

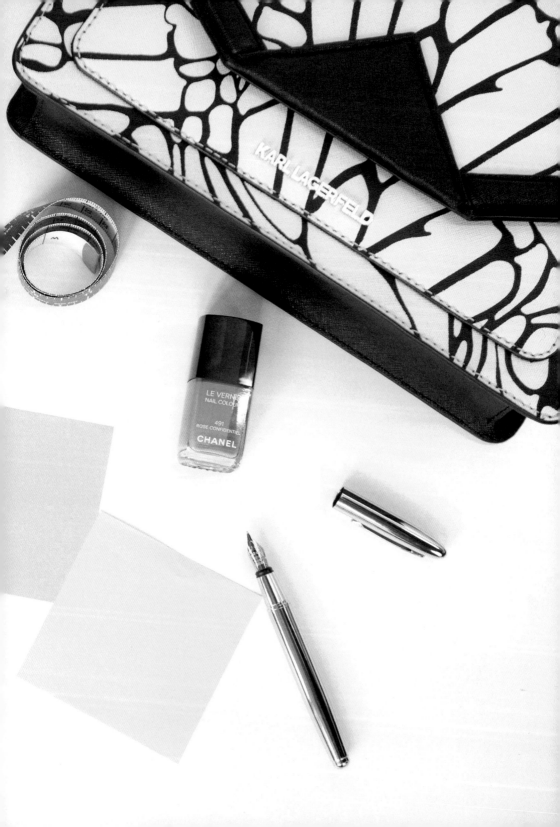

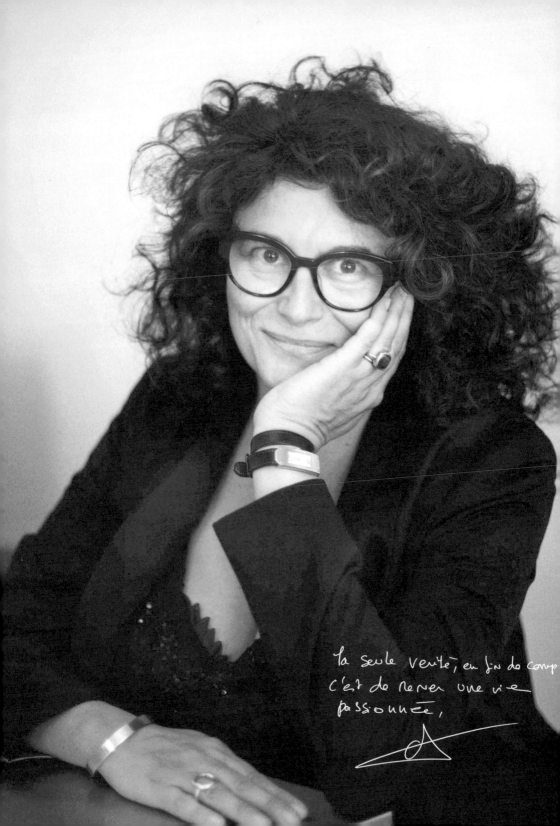

la seule verité, en fin de compte
c'est de mener une vie
passionnée,

Nathalie Cros-Coitton

AGE: 53
PROFESSION: Head of the modeling agency Women
FIRST JOB: Model
YOUR FAVORITE PHOTO OF YOURSELF: A portrait in *Façade*, wearing a leather bustier during the Palace nightclub era in Paris
ASTROLOGICAL SIGN: Leo
DISTINGUISHING FEATURE: Hair and glasses
WHAT CAN'T YOU LIVE WITHOUT: Cell phone and chocolate
WHAT DO YOU DO AS A SPECIAL TREAT FOR YOURSELF: It's a secret (laughter)
YOUR THREE SIGNATURE WARDROBE PIECES: The gorgeous Chloé bag from my agents, my Chaumet wedding ring, and the Vêtements clothes I don't yet own
THREE MUST-HAVE BEAUTY PRODUCTS: Carita's Fluide de Beauté, Rouge G de Guerlain lipstick, Leonor Greyl shampoo
YOUR PERFUME: Guerlain's Eau de Fleurs de Cédrat; Nicolaï's eaux de cologne, Annick Goutal's Eau d'Hadrien
WHO IS YOUR IDOL: All the anonymous women in the world out there fighting for their rights, children, and respect
WHAT BOOK IS ON YOUR NIGHTSTAND: All of Pablo Neruda's books
YOUR LUCKY CHARM: Happiness is something you develop. But I have a box of souvenir photos, letters, notebooks, and small objects from important times in my life.
LESS OR MORE: Both, by turns
YOUR MOTTO: "Never give up."
YOUR ADVICE FOR READERS: To be beautiful, take care of your hair and skin, find the right makeup for you, play with fashion and do your thing with it. Don't try to be someone else, be no-holds-barred daring.

Do you agree that "you only get one chance to make a good impression"? It's better to make a good impression from the start, but if you're smart, you can always get things back on track.
When you meet a model for the first time, what details do you zero in on? I look at her overall figure, her aura. She can have flaws, but what is important at first glance is her demeanor, what she conveys. Next, I look at the cut and color of her hair, and her skin.
Over the course of your career, which model has made the best impression on you and why? That's difficult to answer because I've had several favorites. When I started out, there were Stephanie Seymour, Linda Evangelista, Christy Turlington, and Yasmin Lebon. I came across all the greatest stars of the 1990s because I started in 1985.
A tip for being able to walk like a model? The most important thing is to stand straight, look straight ahead, and don't hesitate.
Does perfection exist? I'm still searching for it...
Three tips for women for improving their chances of making a good impression? I remember an important thing my father used to say to me when I was a child: "You must always have beautiful hair and shoes; if something isn't right in between, it doesn't matter." Personally, I would add a chic handbag to that.

———

Facing page: The only truth, in the end, is to dream of a passionate life.

DAY

02

GETTING ADVICE FROM THE

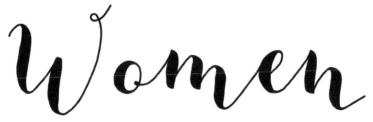

Women

WHO INSPIRE ME

WHERE DO I COME FROM?

THE **MEMORIES** ON WHICH OUR **FOUNDATION** IS BUILT

"**Sisterhood:** the close relationship
among women based
on shared experiences, concerns, etc."

Merriam-Webster

Women have always loved to get together to chat, share ideas, laugh, and give each other advice: it's so much fun! We love to tell each other our secrets over tea, get decked out together for a party, talk about our children if we are mothers, do a group horoscope session, or compare answers to a women's magazine quiz. I love the term that defines female solidarity: sisterhood.

The influential French historian Fernand Braudel once said that "to know where we're going, we must remember where we come from."

We've all grown up among women whose influence helped develop our personality, thus our identity.

From the earliest age we observe the women in our environment in order to develop.

In this chapter we're going to look back in time: who were the women who influenced our childhood? The ones who helped us become who we are. Not just our mother, grandmothers, aunts, or schoolteachers, but also our friends. The women we admire either

for their beauty and style or their ideas. Love them or hate them, these women, who are more or less close to us, have an influence on us throughout our life.

For me, I think about both of my grandmothers. I love watching older women. They guide me along through life. Seeing yourself at every age and projecting yourself into the future is essential. When I was younger I had an idea of what I would be at thirty, and I was so proud once I got there. I will soon be forty-five and by the same token, thanks to my role models, I know exactly what I would like to be at that time. Believe me, there's work to do!

I admired Marie-Andrée for her warmth, vanilla-scented creams, elegance, refinement, beautiful white hair, and powdery perfumes. Until the end (she died at age 93), when I would visit her in her rest home, she always greeted me with her hair done and wearing pretty clothes: such a great joy! Seeing her that way gave me hope and strength.

I like to think, like Françoise Giroud— French writer and cofounder of the magazine *Marie Claire* with Jean Prouvost—that

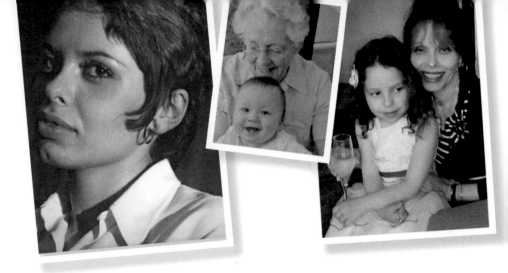

Left to right: Christel's mother, her grandmother Marie-Andrée,
and her daughter Lilo with Christel's mother.

"taking care of yourself" is a duty, a kind of politeness toward others. In an interview for *Elle*, Cécilia Attias, ex-wife of former French president Nicolas Sarkozy, recalled her Russian grandmother's motto: "hold on and hold up." Worth remembering when life is not so sweet.

I get my blue eyes from Jeannine, my other grandma who is still alive. Jeannine is from a working-class milieu, and she always bravely fought her way through hard times. Once when we were in the bathroom, getting ourselves ready to go to the cemetery to bury my grandfather, she said to me: "Make the most of every moment, my little sweetie, life goes by so fast." I think of it often.

Women's relationships consist of con-nections and sharing. Jeannine is the one who gave my mother *Le Livre du Bonheur* by Marcelle Auclair, which translates as "The Book of Happiness," which I still have and will one day pass on to my own daughter. It's just the kind of book we like, filled with recipes for good living.

When French actress Fanny Ardant was asked in an interview, "What do you think you have handed down to your daughters?" she answered, "An independence of spirit, I think. To be incorrigible. A child must learn that life is full of risks, but you have to take them. I always told them, 'Choose, choose which side you're on' … and 'find a passion, money doesn't matter, nor does success. What matters is waking up in the morning thinking you wouldn't trade places with anyone.' I never asked them to be happy, but intense. When you're intense, even misfortune passes quickly."

Obviously my mother inspired me a lot: she is a kind of Betty Boop with short black hair (is that why I always wanted long hair?). I remember her look in the 1980s—stilettos, leather mini-skirt, trendy red lipstick—con-trasted with that of my classmates' mothers, who wore classic clothes and flats. At the time, I thought my mother was too focused on being fashionable, yet today I've adopted the same style!

24

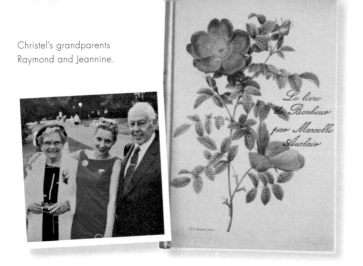

Christel's grandparents
Raymond and Jeannine.

CREATING OUR BENCHMARKS

I t is just so important to have friends to share our ideas with—our ideas about life, men, children, and clothes!

I'm lucky to have the same friends I've had since I was a teenager: my friend Karyn is small like me and she's my kindred spirit. She has always fascinated me because she is rigorous and loyal. Then there's Sara, who's tall and dynamic; conversations with her are a delight.

These two women are both very different from me, and I love listening to them and observing them, because it gives me energy.

Figuring out your look by watching others and gleaning inspiration from the past through family photos is great fun! Now it's your turn to observe the people in your entourage, past and present. It can be a woman you saw in the office lobby whose energy and aura made a huge impact on you or an elderly person with incredible style—anyone from a passing inspiration to the role model of a lifetime.

Delve into your family albums, dive into your memories, and pick out, as I did, the women who counted and still count for you. Do the work of remembering and do your research: who are the women who carried you through, the women you admire?

Who do you look like? Who do you not wish to look like? That's just as important: having counter-idols—looks and people you don't like at all—strengthens your values and the idea you have of yourself. Also think about what you've picked up from the men in your family. In an interview with *Marie-Claire*, the fabulous French actress Céline Sallette revealed the following: "Femininity, in my family, comes from my dad's side—and it's very rural and earthy."

DAY
02

INSPIRATION TREE

All you need are reference points
to advance in life! Paste your photo
memories here of your friends
and family who inspire you.
Where do you fit into the picture?

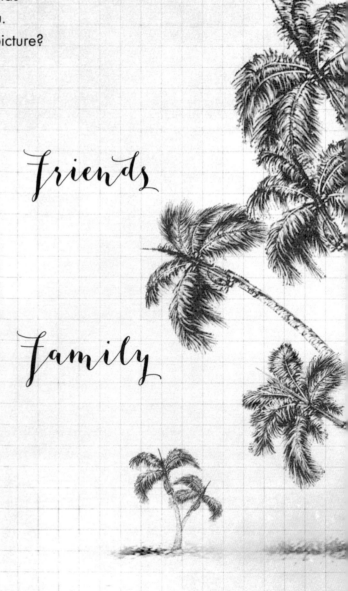

Friends

Family

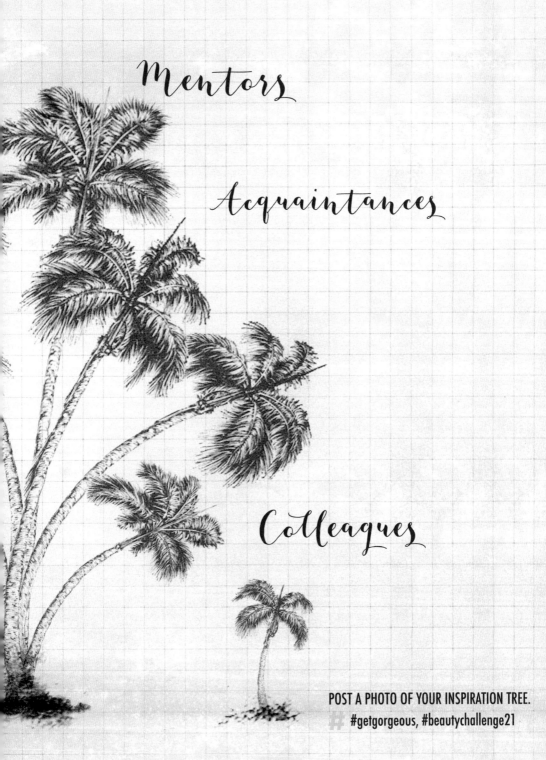

Mentors

Acquaintances

Colleagues

POST A PHOTO OF YOUR INSPIRATION TREE.
#getgorgeous, #beautychallenge21

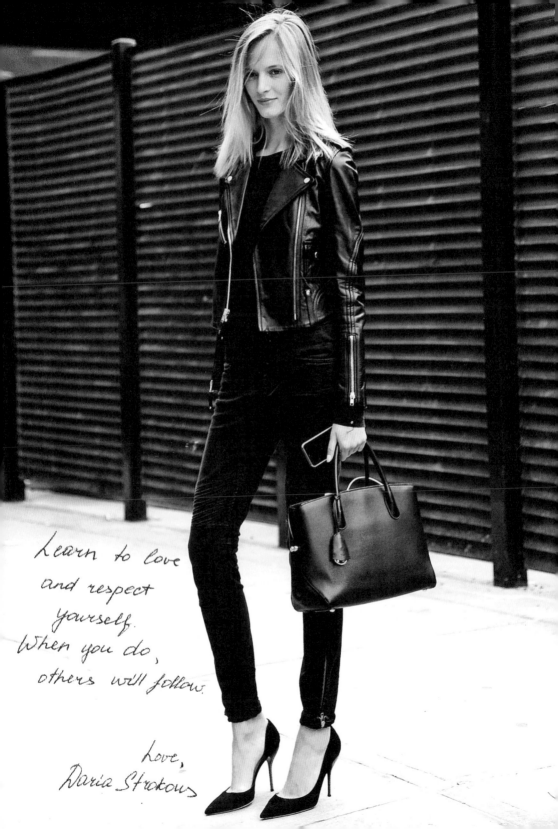

Learn to love
and respect
yourself.
When you do,
others will follow.

Love,
Daria Strokous

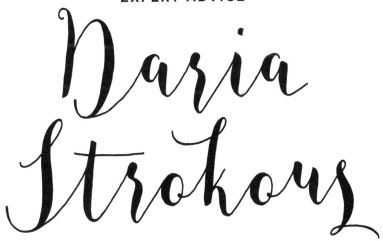

Daria Strokous

AGE: 26
DISTINGUISHING FEATURE: Blue and yellow eyes
ASTROLOGICAL SIGN: Libra
PROFESSION: Model
FIRST JOB: Prada S/S '08 show
YOUR FAVORITE PHOTO OF YOURSELF: One
of me with my dad when I was little
YOUR LUCKY CHARM: I always carry a string bracelet
that my sister brought back for me from Tibet
WHAT BOOK IS ON YOUR NIGHTSTAND:
Right now it's *Mythology 101*
WHAT CAN'T YOU LIVE WITHOUT: Dessert!
WHO IS YOUR IDOL: Audrey Hepburn
YOUR THREE SIGNATURE WARDROBE PIECES:
Leather jacket, over-the-knee boots, mini skirt
THREE MUST-HAVE BEAUTY PRODUCTS: Biologique
Recherche moisturizer, Homéoplasmine® (gel
to soothe skin irritations), coconut oil
YOUR PERFUME: I change it occasionally, but it's
always something with notes of sandalwood
LESS OR MORE: Less
WHAT DO YOU DO AS A SPECIAL TREAT
FOR YOURSELF: I get lots of sweets,
chocolate, and ice-cream and eat it all while
binge-watching a good new TV show
YOUR MOTTO: "Every problem has a solution."
YOUR ADVICE FOR READERS: Learn to love and
respect yourself. When you do, others will follow.

What woman inspired you as a child? My
godmother, Nina. She has always looked perfect.
Styled hair and perfect makeup, red nail polish
and red lipstick, no matter where you saw
her. And always optimistic. A true lady.
Who is your favorite fictional heroine? Catherine
Tramell (Sharon Stone's character in *Basic Instinct*).
Are you more Blondie, Patti Smith, or Cher? Cher.
She is an example of a confident woman who is
not afraid to express her style. Plus, I love dressing
up and dancing to pop oldies and disco music.
Who do you wish you looked like? Michelle
Pfeiffer in *Scarface*, when I go out.
What have you learned from your friends?
All our experiences shape who we are. So
don't judge the people around you, you might
understand them much better with time.
Should icons be taken off their pedestal? I think
icons should be on pedestals, but we have to be
very careful when choosing who we put up there.

DAY

03

MAKING MY

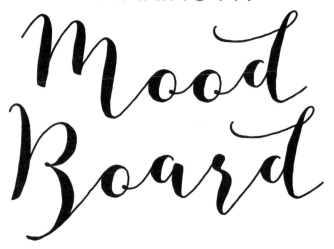

MY INSPIRATIONS

WHAT IS A **MOOD BOARD**, ANYWAY?

A mood board, a visually inspiring wall, is a creative tool designers, graphics artists, and photographers use for displaying the trends and inspirations behind their work.

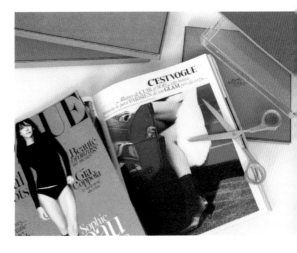

In early childhood we create the image of our ideal self. We do this at first through contact with the women around us (*see* Day 2). After that, we turn to characters in novels, celebrities, actresses, singers, and models for inspiration.

What kind of woman do you want to be? Who do you want to be like? In all honesty, you know who you are now. Using your mood board you are going to define the woman you dream of becoming.

A mood board is like a poster (physical or digital) where you assemble various images, colors, words, and materials to "tell a story" and develop a theme.

I've always been drawn to visual groupings that remind me of artists' collages, like photographer Peter Beard's travel notes. When I was working for *Numéro* magazine, such walls of images fascinated me.

Well before then, in the 1990s—the golden age of top models—I started making my first collages in my bedroom as a teenager. It was my way of appropriating all those glossy paper images that sometimes felt a bit distant, of making them my own by playing around with them. It was my way of putting my foot into the still-closed doors of the FASHION world.

TODAY I'M GOING **TO HELP** YOU **MAKE** YOUR OWN **MOOD BOARD**

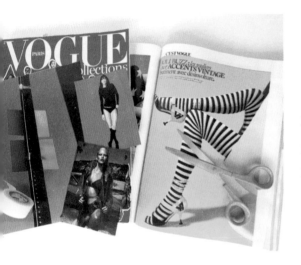

Don't be afraid, go for it, no one else is listening, we're all women here!

I see myself long ago, daydreaming as I leafed through my grandmother's magazines in the attic when I was a young girl. Back then, the first issues of *Elle* and the drawings in an old French fashion weekly for women called *Petit Echo de la Mode*—with its retro figures and the fine, neat, stylish clothes the models wore—inspired me.

The actress Jeanne Moreau was one of the first to have awakened the curious, pleasant feeling of attraction in me. Everything about her fascinated me: her wonderful blondness of course, her husky voice, her demeanor—a mix of feminine pride and sensuality. This adoration was confirmed a few years later when I crossed paths with her for the first time. I asked, "What is your secret?", and she scribbled the following on a piece of paper for me: "A piece of advice, which? Love yourself!"

My second idol was Renée Simonsen, a supermodel ahead of her time and engaged to John Taylor, Duran Duran's guitarist. For me she was the perfect woman, the one I dreamed of looking like. With a mass of blond hair, Renée embodied the American-style, healthy girl look (even though she's actually

You'll see, your mood board will turn out to be of precious help, a sort of guide to the things that inspire you, an ally that will help you find your inner fashion model.

It's time to whip out the scissors and glue and your favorite photos and images.

The first step involves collecting a certain number of images. To help with your research, I encourage you to get creative by answering one simple question: who are the women, models, actresses, singers, artists, novelists, and female politicians who fascinate you the most, those you would really like to resemble? To put it simply, who are your IDOLS?

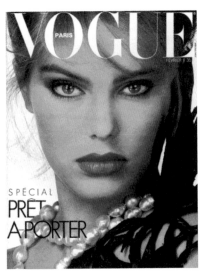

Renée Simonsen.

Danish). She had fabulous curves, slender legs, a tiny waist, aerodynamic breasts, a harmoniously structured face with a perfect complexion, full lips, and big blue eyes. She was my childhood Barbie doll in the flesh.

I grew up under the influence of these two blonds, guided by two extreme visions of women: on one side the sculpted, almost unreal perfection of the model; and on the other side the actress and her weaknesses, whose influence on me was both physical and intellectual.

un conseil le quel ? Aimez-vous !

Jeanne Moreau

YOUR **MOOD BOARD** CAN INCLUDE:

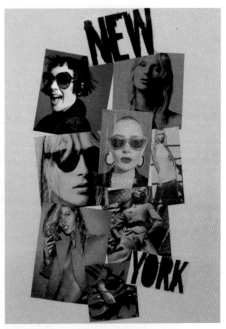

- Images of the celebrities who **inspire** you (actresses, actors, models, notable people of all kinds, etc.)
- **Atmospheric** photos (interiors, exteriors, places, or objects)
- **Words, quotes**
- **Materials** (papers, fabrics, wood, etc.)
- **Colors**
- **Drawings** (your own, as well)
- **Everything you like** and that moves you

"ONE IS NOT BORN A WOMAN BUT BECOMES ONE."

SIMONE DE BEAUVOIR

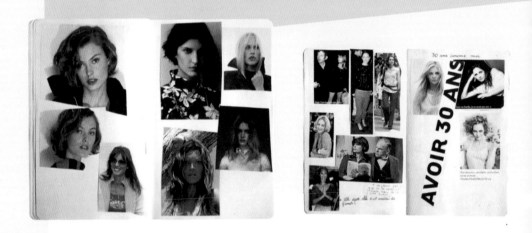

HOW DO YOU ACTUALLY GO ABOUT **FINDING IMAGES?**

Whether or not you're the type to hang onto things, or whether or not you love clipping photos from magazines, don't worry. Today, you can find everything you need on the Internet. Personally, I recommend pinterest.com, which is very handy for creating mood boards and where it's easy to search for images using keywords (colors, names of models, photographs, etc.). The advantage this site has over Google images is that you can find so many quality visuals. You can also check out tumblr.com.

Now it's your turn to make a **LIST OF THE WOMEN** who make you dream.

03

....

....

....

....

....

....

....

Next let's start the research work, which will help you illustrate your vision of the ideal woman and shape it onto your mood board.

At this stage in the process of creating your board, don't censure yourself: look through your favorite books and magazines, collect everything you can think of—photos, drawings, and even words and quotes. Once you have all your visuals together, scatter them on the board so that you can have a good overall view.

I love doing this exercise using paper images. It's more concrete.

It's time for you to sort through the images you feel are related to one another and that have more of a story to tell. Try to keep only about ten of the best ones, the ones that you like 100%.

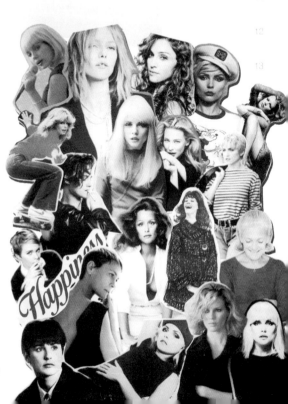

35

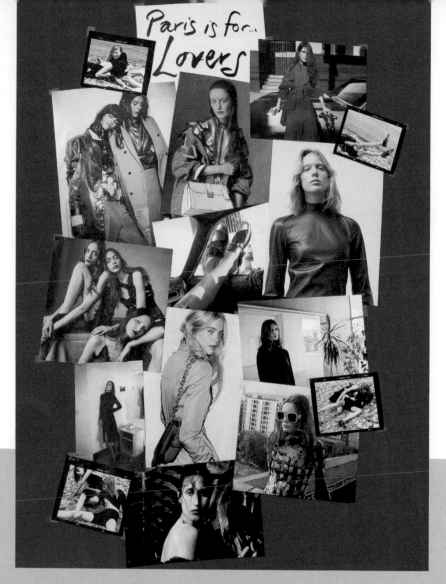

Paris is for... *Lovers*

I t's time to assemble your mood board. If you've chosen paper, glue the images onto solid, large-format Bristol board (as I did for mine) or construction paper. The order doesn't matter much. Do as you like, and don't hesitate to draw on it, if you like, or to add some of your key words with a marker. If you prefer the Internet, check out my Pinterest page and you'll see how I organized mine.

Finally if you don't want to share it with everyone, you can keep the identity of your ideal woman a secret, slipping it in between the pages, here.

A DETAILED
PORTRAIT

Jot down the features
of your **IDEAL WOMAN**
here; they'll become
your **KEY WORDS**.

You now have a clear view of the woman who inspires you, the one you dream of being. Beyond this or that celebrity, you are now able to make out the woman's features, to define a kind of identikit of this ideal: her face, look, demeanor, etc.

For me she is clearly blond, has red lips, blue eyes, and always wears heels—which doesn't stop me from liking men's shirts and jackets.

What about your idol? What does she look like?

Be proud of yourself, because even though it can seem a little abstract, the work you've just done is essential for the rest of this twenty-one day challenge. You have just laid the foundations for YOUR STYLE, the one my friends say is so difficult to find!

POST YOUR MOOD BOARD.
\# #getgorgeous, #beautychallenge21

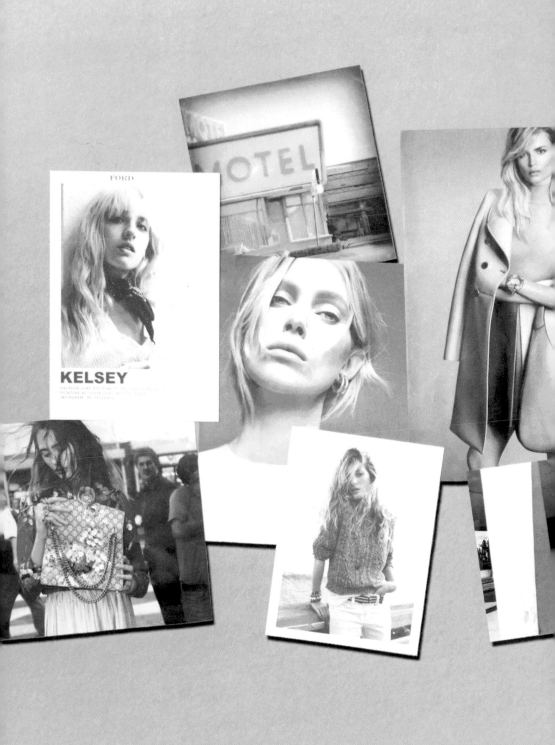

FORD

KELSEY

MOTEL

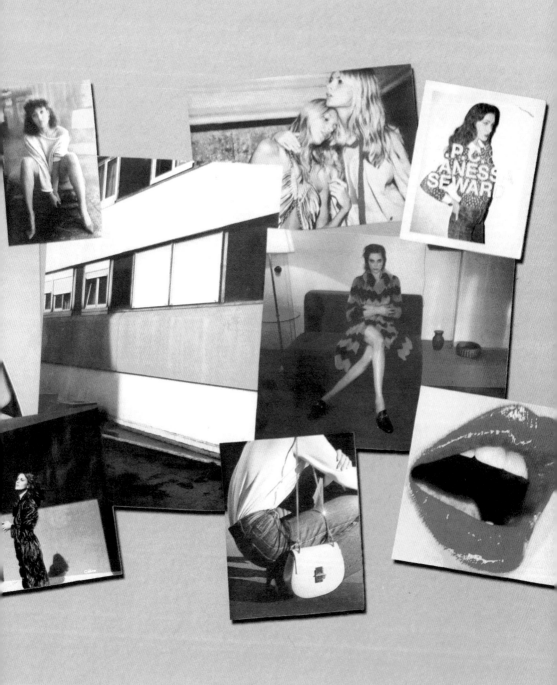

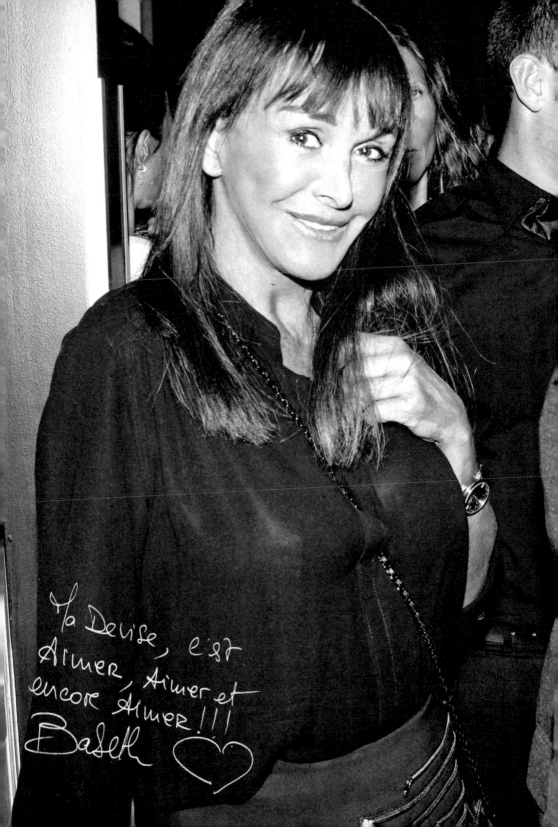

Ma Devise, c'est
Aimer, Aimer et
encore Aimer !!!
Baseth ♡

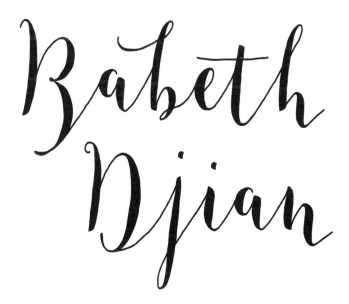

Babeth Djian

AGE: 25!!
PROFESSION: Editor in chief of *Numéro* magazine and *Numéro Homme*
FIRST JOB: Cofounder of the magazine *Jill* (jillmag.fr)
YOUR FAVORITE PHOTO OF YOURSELF: A shot of me by Peter Lindbergh at Coney Island in 1990
ASTROLOGICAL SIGN: Cancer with Leo ascendant
DISTINGUISHING FEATURE: Laughter
WHAT CAN'T YOU LIVE WITHOUT: Love
WHAT DO YOU DO AS A SPECIAL TREAT FOR YOURSELF: I'm a gourmand
YOUR THREE SIGNATURE WARDROBE PIECES: Black, black, and black
THREE MUST-HAVE BEAUTY PRODUCTS: My smile
YOUR PERFUME: Orange blossom; I was born in Morocco
WHO IS YOUR IDOL: My friends
WHAT BOOK IS ON YOUR NIGHTSTAND: *La Puissance de la joie* (the power of joy) by Frédéric Lenoir
YOUR LUCKY CHARM: My snake
LESS OR MORE: More! I'm unfamiliar with less.
YOUR MOTTO (facing page): "Love, love, and love some more."
YOUR ADVICE FOR READERS: Live every moment intensely; live in the present.

Are you for or against mood boards? Neither for nor against, I go by my intuition.
Do you use paper or digital mood boards? Either one, it's just a work tool.
What advice can you offer readers for making their first mood board? Follow your heart.
What things inspire you (cinema, music, contemporary art, deco, etc.)? Everything inspires me, even a bad film.
Do you keep your mood boards? I don't keep anything.
Who are your fashion icons? My friend for life, Jean Paul Gaultier, who helped me win first prize at Studio Berçot; thanks to him I started this career. The old and the new generation, in alphabetical order: Alber Elbaz, Bouchra Jarrar, Demna Gvasalia, Haider Ackermann, Hedi Slimane, Karl Lagerfeld, Rick Owens. And I'm forgetting some!
Are you for or against the current cult of images? Neither for nor against, I like images!

DAY

04

GETTING DOWN TO THE

Basics

MY ESSENTIALS

WHAT EXACTLY IS A **BASIC**?

"**Basics,** also called 'musts,' are key items of clothing that blend style and function. Brands and labels stick with them every season, in new colors or fabrics, with a new detail or length."

Catherine Bézard

A wardrobe basic, contrary to what the word indicates, isn't necessarily an overly simple, inexpensive piece of clothing, it's one that's essential to your wardrobe. What your look centers around.

We call it a "must-have" and that's a well-chosen term. In reality a basic is the item you must possess at all costs. It's a real chameleon in your closet. You can wear it in the evening or the daytime, on vacation or on the job.

Basics are easy to spot yet coming up with an exhaustive list of them is almost impossible. Culture and setting also come into play. A New Yorker's basic is not necessarily the same for a Parisian or Londoner. What's most important is for you to be able to pick out YOURS.

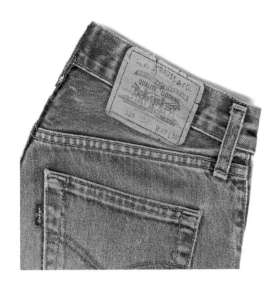

WHAT ARE YOUR
BASICS?

Here are a few tricks
for helping you identify them.

1 YOU **ALWAYS WANT TO BUY IT** AGAIN AFTER YOU'VE WORN IT TO DEATH
This is surely the best criterion of all. We all know what it's like when our jeans have become too threadbare to be worn in public and yet we just can't bring ourselves to throw them out. That's when it's time to buy a new pair!

2 IT ALWAYS GETS YOU **COMPLIMENTS**
You know very well which one I mean. For me it's the little 1950s number, the cotton dress with the buttons, Peter Pan collar, and cinched waist, which I have in at least six different colors. Trust your memory. Some clothes get you lots more compliments than others, don't they? When I say compliments I mean it makes heads turn. You have to be careful about compliments from "fake friends" who say things like, "That looks so great on you, only you could ever wear it." The true compliment is often the absence of one with a tight-lipped look followed by a purchase identical to yours in the next few days.

3 YOU FEEL **PERFECTLY COMFORTABLE** WEARING IT
Sometimes style is the enemy of comfort (more on this later, *see* Day 14), but wearing only uncomfortable clothes and accessories is inconceivable.

Often men's opinion of what's feminine does not spell comfort, which is why it took a woman, Coco Chanel, to get women out of their corsets. The benefit you get from clothes perfectly suited to your body is just as wonderful as the benefit from a more spectacular and necessarily confining look.

Feeling at ease does not mean looking sloppy, it's about the perfect harmony of a jacket whose cut is flattering to your figure without weighing it down, or a pair of four-inch heels you can walk around in all day. For example I don't like the jogging or sweatpants look—it is too sloppy and it flatters absolutely nothing. I agree with Karl Lagerfeld: "Sweatpants are an admission of failure. You've lost control of your life when you've bought a pair of sweatpants."

The idea of comfort simply indicates to you that an item of clothing is tailor made for you, that it's your "must-have."

"EVERYONE CAN DRESS CHIC AND GLAMOROUS FOR AN EVENING, BUT IT'S HOW PEOPLE DRESS EVERY DAY THAT IS THE MOST FASCINATING."

ALEXANDER WANG

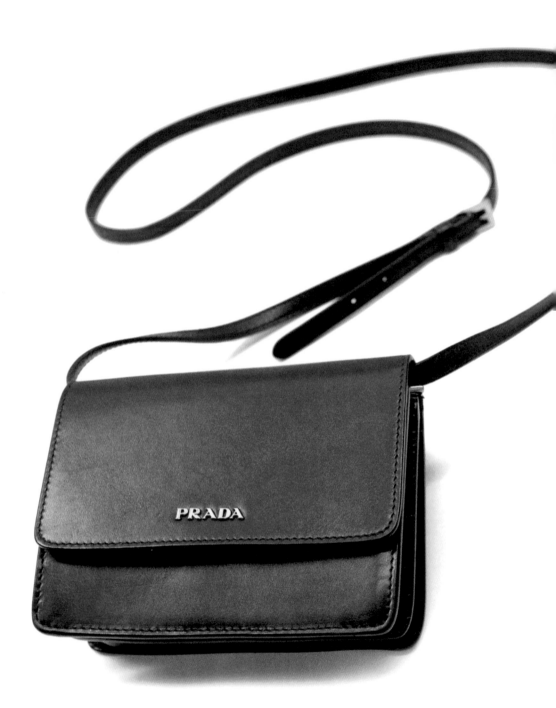

4 THE COLOR **GOES WITH ALMOST EVERYTHING**

Again, Coco Chanel once said, "The most beautiful color of all is the one that looks good on you."

I'll never say it enough: there is no set recipe, only PERSONAL solutions to each of these issues. Obviously, you naturally expect a basic to have a basic color, right? But if pink is your favorite color, go for it!

In general, white, gray, navy, denim blue, and black are the five real pillars of any wardrobe. Except for certain classic patterns such as gingham, sailor stripes, or Scottish plaids, the word basic often refers to solid colors, without patterns, making the basic article infinitely combinable with clothes of brighter and more complementary colors.

For the pickiest perfectionists, having only basics of the same color would be ideal. This way they could practically dress in the dark and not make a mistake. In fact there is a term for this. It's a real science, where you come up with a total look in one single color that shades off into several different tones.

5 IT OUTLASTS **TIMES AND TRENDS**

In short, basics are clothes that last. Of course they're of good quality and are not necessarily expensive but are solid, like jeans, or, on the contrary, delicate and more luxurious with impeccable details, like the Hermès Kelly bag.

The fabric used for basics is key and usually natural—a beautiful cotton canvas, thick leather, 8-ply cashmere, or superb silk chiffon.

The cut is every bit as basic, rather simple, without fancy flourishes, effective. The ideal cut for a basic is the one that a woman of any age could wear.

Sometimes brands try and make us believe that a certain new bag is a real must-have. Remember when it-bags were all the rage a few years ago? I would tend to say, "wait and see," giving it another ten or fifteen years.

REMINDER: IT'S A **BASIC** IF

- You **always** want to **buy it again**
- It always gets you **compliments**
- You feel **perfectly comfortable** wearing it
- The **color goes with** almost **everything**
- It **outlasts** times and trends

CHRISTEL'S **BASICS**

You'll notice my basics are a mix of cheap and chic clothes. I've worn some of them since I was fifteen. I'm not obsessed with brands, but, over time, I have learned to invest a little money in certain beautiful items. If you can treat yourself to them, they'll last a lifetime!

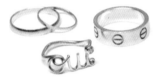

Accessories

- Aviator sunglasses (Ray Ban)
- Maxi sunglasses with slightly tinted lenses (Isabel Marant or from street markets)
- Black sunglasses with acetate frames (Persol)
- Men's round watch with leather strap (Patek Philippe, or your boyfriend's)
- Rings, bracelets, and thin gold chains (any that are simple, minimalist, and 100% gold)
- Natural leather belt, square buckle (Chloé or vintage)
- Tote bag (Louis Vuitton or canvas)
- Clutch (Olympia Le-Tan or & Other Stories)
- Scarf (Hermès or vintage bandanna)

Tops

- Loose-fitting cream-colored shirt (in silk at Equipment, viscose at Zara)
- White cotton, crew neck T-shirt (Prada or Fruit of the Loom)
- Silk lingerie top with thin straps and lace details (La Perla or Victoria's Secret)
- Man's white cotton shirt with thin blue stripes (Dior Homme or Uniqlo)
- Flecked gray cotton sweatshirt (APC or Asos)
- Navy blue V-neck cashmere pullover (Hermès or Gap)
- Cotton sailor shirt (Isabel Marant Étoile or Agnès B.)

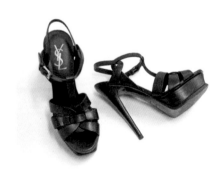

Shirts & dresses

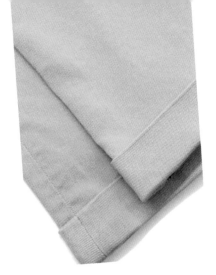

- Black cocktail dress (Victoria Beckham or Zara)
- Cotton shirtdress (APC or vintage)
- Jean skirt (APC or Levi's®)

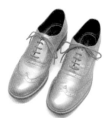

Pants

- Straight-cut, high-waist raw denim jeans (Chloé or Levi's®)
- Light gray skinny jeans (Cheap Monday or H&M)
- Men's pleated pants in cotton canvas or wool (Haider Ackermann or Uniqlo)
- Camel-colored cotton chinos (Ralph Lauren or Zara)

Shoes

- Pointy 3-inch low-cut heels (Gianvito Rossi or Asos)
- Dizzyingly high heels (Saint Laurent Tribute or nothing)
- Derbies (Church's or Clarks)
- Ballerina flats (Repetto or Zara)
- Canvas high-tops (Converse® and nothing else)

Jackets & coats

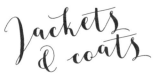

- Men's straight-cut wool coat (Jil Sander or Cos)
- Loose-fitting navy-blue blazer (Pallas or J.Crew)
- The adjustable-fit leather motorcycle jacket (Acne Studios or vintage)
- Tobacco-colored trench coat (Burberry or vintage)

Other

- Button-down cotton jumpsuit (APC or Asos)
- Denim shorts (vintage or homemade)

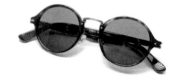

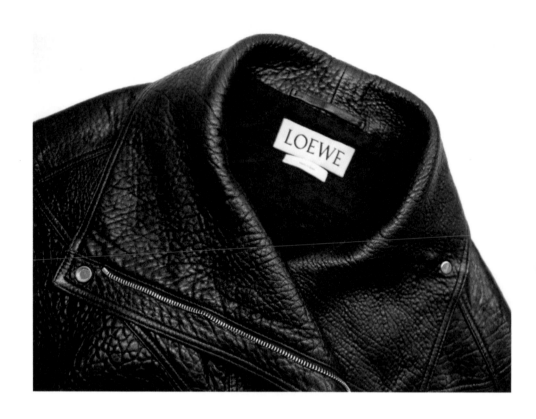

Here's a little trick you can do:
have fun taking photos of your basics
with a real Polaroid or your smartphone.
Paste your photos here
or pin them up in your closet.
It's one way to be sure you don't
forget about any of your clothes.

DAY
04

Now it's your turn
to make your own list of *your* basics!

....
....
....
....
....
....
....
....
....
....
....
....
....
....
....
....
....

POST A PHOTO OF YOUR FAVORITE BASICS.
#getgorgeous, #beautychallenge21

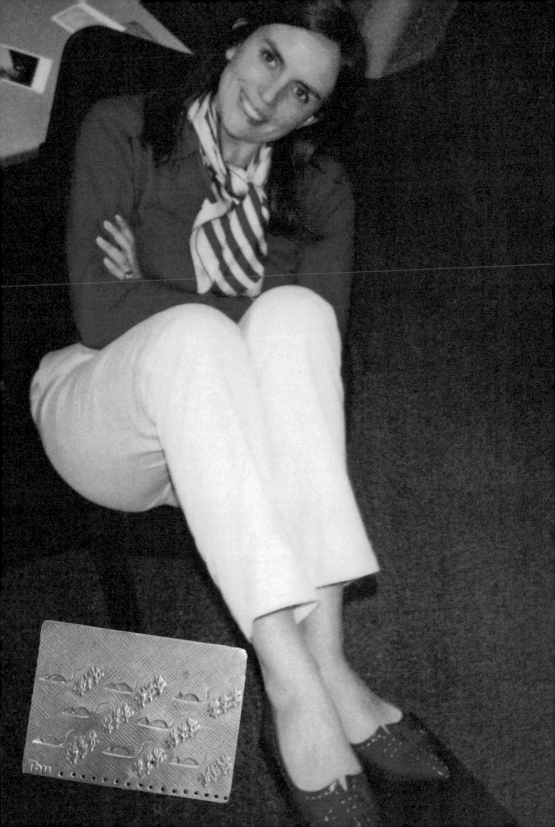

Priscille d'Orgeval

AGE: 50
PROFESSION: Fashion editor, stylist
FIRST JOB: Nicole Crassat's[1] assistant
YOUR FAVORITE PHOTO OF YOURSELF:
A portrait of a man by August Sander
ASTROLOGICAL SIGN: Gemini
DISTINGUISHING FEATURE: I cross the city by bicycle
WHAT CAN'T YOU LIVE WITHOUT: Tea
WHAT DO YOU DO AS A SPECIAL TREAT
FOR YOURSELF: Ride my bike along the
Seine, past the *bouquiniste* kiosks
YOUR THREE SIGNATURE WARDROBE
PIECES: An old tuxedo shirt, a pair of APC
jeans, and my Church's derbies
THREE MUST-HAVE BEAUTY PRODUCTS:
Santa Maria Novella's aromatic waters, Leonor
Greyl's Shampooing Crème Moelle de Bambou,
and Elizabeth Arden's Eight Hour Cream
YOUR PERFUME: Guerlain's L'Heure Bleue
in winter and Santa Maria Novella's eau
de cologne Zagara in summer
WHO IS YOUR IDOL: Diane Keaton and Jerry Hall
WHAT BOOK IS ON YOUR NIGHTSTAND:
Snoopy and cookbooks
YOUR LUCKY CHARM: Twelve thin gold and
silver bangles that I've worn for thirty years
LESS OR MORE: Neither more nor
less, just enough for me
YOUR MOTTO: "Smile, always smile."
YOUR ADVICE FOR READERS: Have fun!

Cheap or chic basics? Cheap.
Men's shirt or white T-shirt? Men's shirt.
Jeans or pleated trousers? Jeans.
Heels or derbies? Derbies.
Sunglasses on or off? On.
You never go without...? A scarf.
Favorite color? Sky blue.
Where do you buy wardrobe basics?
At APC, Uniqlo, or flea markets.

———

[1.] Nicolle Grassat was a highly respected stylist
in the fashion world who worked at *Elle* magazine
for about ten years and supported young designers
who later became famous, including Azzedine Alaïa
and Jean Paul Gaultier.

DAY

05

EDITING MY

Wardrobe

ORGANIZE MY CLOSET

CLEAR OUT THE **CLUTTER**, **NO REGRETS**

"I'm like every other woman:
a closet full of clothes,
but nothing to wear—so I wear jeans."

Cameron Diaz

Let's get down to the nitty-gritty. As you'll have seen by now, this book is not about selling you illusions, it's about creating a link between your fashion reality and fashion dreams. Bridging this gap is entirely possible, and it starts with the basics. The next step is to dive into your private world by rummaging through your closet.

Some of you will tell yourselves: "But I don't have a walk-in closet. At most I have an old armoire where I try to organize my clothes." I assure you, neither do I, and I know few women who have a real walk-in closet.

Yet we shouldn't totally abandon the idea of having a famous walk-in closet like the character Carrie Bradshaw had in *Sex & the City*, should we?

This mysterious room, a real fashion treasure trove of clothes is in reality a symbolic place for a woman. The walk-in closet is the descendant of the eighteenth-century boudoir so well described by the Marquis de Sade in *Philosophy in the Bedroom:* it's a place, with its rituals and furniture, dressing table and mirror, its drawers filled with little secrets we don't always want to share.

Whether you have a simple armoire or a real walk-in closet, what you have to do is the same: you just have to find a space, as small as it might be, that's yours and yours alone.

It goes without saying that if you don't have either an armoire or a drawer all to yourself, it's time to shake things up at home. I love sharing my space with my fiancé and my three children, but everything has a limit; I like the idea of having my own "territory" just for me. Without it, it would be hard for me to maintain my identity as a woman.

LET'S **GET TO WORK**!

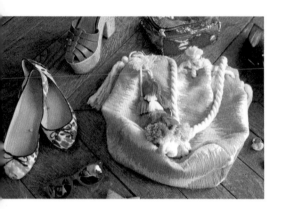

1 OPERATION **CLOSET CLEAN-OUT** (START OVER FROM SCRATCH)

My technique for revamping my closet is very simple and it consists of only one thing: throwing things out. I know it can be painful to get rid of the old clothes you love. But be realistic, how many mornings have you stood with a desperate look as you faced your closet yelling: "I DON'T HAVE ANYTHING TO WEAR!"?

Ok, you always end up finding the right clothes, but often at the cost of getting seriously upset and wasting time.

Let's avoid that! We're a bit foggy when we first wake up. Asking our brain to find a top that goes with a pair of pants, which itself must go with a pair of shoes, all lying in a heap—some of which are clean and ironed and others which have been worn, but it's hard to distinguish which is which—that's just impossible!

So today let's take the time—and the luxury—to wipe the slate clean of our bad habits and put an end to "closet panic."

Empty out your entire closet. And I mean empty. Entirely! Lay out all your clothes and accessories on your bed. Don't worry, we're going to look at all of them.

2 OPERATION **MAKEOVER** (GIVE YOUR CLOSET A SILVER LINING)

Before starting to sort your clothes, look at the empty closet. Let's freshen it up a bit and turn this "panic room" into a comfortable, pleasant place. It's time to do this, without breaking the bank.

Invest in a few wooden hangers (they are more gentle on clothes, and don't deform clothes as much as plastic or metal hangers), cover the walls of your closet with fabric or wallpaper or simply paint them in that wonderful color you love that your boyfriend has always vetoed for the living room walls.

In a word, this is your space: invest in it, make yourself happy, don't hesitate to scent it with essential oils, or to pin up a few images that you like—why not your mood board, for example? Personally I always loved the inside of those high-school lockers you see across America and in films, covered with images and little sayings....

Operation closet makeover: DONE!

"THE MOST
BEAUTIFUL
CLOTHES THAT
CAN DRESS A WOMAN
ARE THE ARMS
OF THE MAN
SHE LOVES.
BUT FOR THOSE
WHO HAVEN'T HAD
THE FORTUNE
OF FINDING
THIS HAPPINESS,
I AM THERE."

YVES SAINT LAURENT

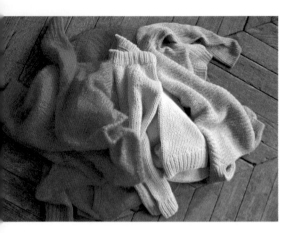

Our aim is to keep only the pieces that potentially go together. Guaranteed to boost your style, while saving time and money.

Like Karl Lagerfeld, top designers and stylists are resolutely faithful to their look, which sometimes veers towards looking like a uniform; that's our aim.

But we're not finished. We're going to repeat the same operation with the clothes that are too old to be perked up and those that are no longer your size. Let's be realistic—when was the last time you wore those size 0 jeans? Summer 2005? Ok, you know what to do.

Ditto for the jacket that you bought too small in the sales, telling yourself "in any case I'll go on a diet in the spring." Get rid of it. If you really lose weight by spring, you deserve to buy a new jacket in your size!

The only exception to the rule is that really beautiful piece that you tell yourself is going to come back in style. While experience dictates that this rarely happens, it's not too important because you are allowed ONE exception.

3 OPERATION **LESS IS MORE** (ORGANIZE, IDENTIFY, CLEAR OUT)

Let's sort through our wardrobe so that it's clearer, visually.

To do so, start by organizing all the clothes by families of color, ditto for accessories.

Logically the dominant colors should appear. If this isn't the case, you are up the creek. Just kidding. As for me, I have my pile of pink (my favorite color), denim blue, white, navy, gray, and black. So far, so good. Strangely I'm unable to put this green sweater into any of my piles.

Surely you see where I'm heading with this, because apart from one flashy accessory that would perk up a monochromatic look, it is time to say goodbye to what I call the "UFOs" in your wardrobe. These false friends, which sometimes have huge sentimental value to you, are only troublemakers that keep you from seeing clearly.

You are free to give them away, donate them to a thrift store or charity organization, or resell them. The main thing is to get rid of them! It can't be said often enough: LESS IS MORE.

4 OPERATION **FRESH START** (BEING GOOD TO YOUR WARDROBE)

You tell yourself the moment has finally come to completely reorganize your beautiful clean closet. Uh, well no actually, that would be too easy.

Take advantage of the moment to pay close attention to the survivors of our closet-organizing session.

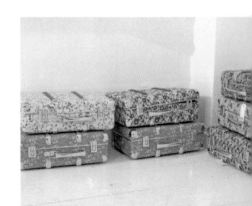

ITEMS THAT WILL HELP
STRAIGHTEN UP YOUR CLOSET:

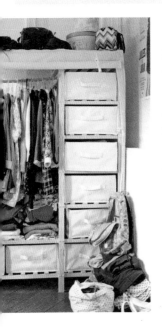

- A garbage bag—to gather the **discard pile**
- Bright fabric, **photos**, paint, post-it notes, your mood board—whatever you want to use to personalize your closet
- Wooden **hangers**
- Garment bags for delicates
- An iron or a steamer
- A **sewing kit**

You have kept the best items from your wardrobe. The happy few deserve to be carefully reviewed: you might need to re-sew the button that's about to fall off your blazer, buy a garment bag to protect your jackets, smooth out the cashmere sweater that is covered in pills, carefully iron the rather wrinkled chinos. We always forget that ironing is an art that can save lots of clothes. If you are no good at it or are short on time, there's always the dry-cleaners: a great idea.

Any clothing designer will tell you that everything comes down to the details; we'll look into this a little further on. In this age of overconsumption, let's buy less but take better care of our clothes; this really makes all the difference.

THERE, YOUR CLOSET IS ORGANIZED:
LET'S SEE HOW IT LOOKS. SHARE A PHOTO.
**#getgorgeous, #beautychallenge21**

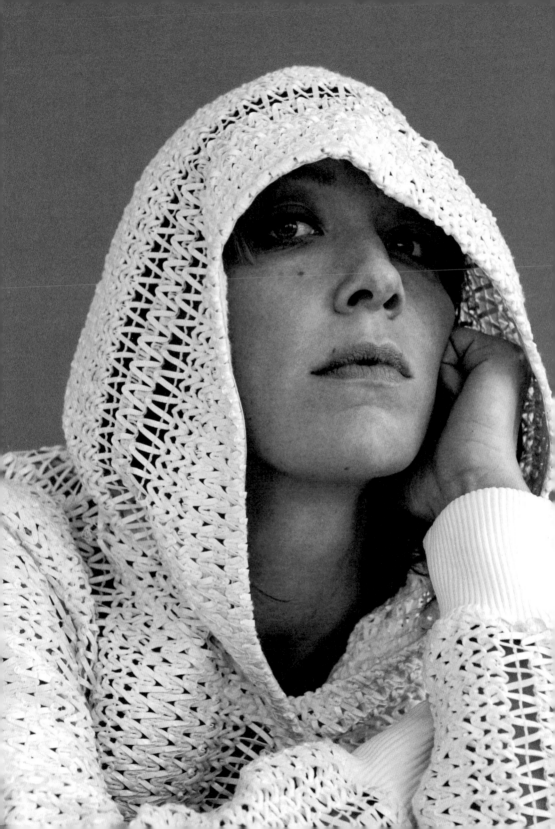

Johanna Senyk

AGE: 33
PROFESSION: Wanda Nylon designer
and creative director
FIRST JOB: Photo stylist
YOUR FAVORITE PHOTO OF YOURSELF: A photo of
myself when I was little, milking a cow in Poland
ASTROLOGICAL SIGN: Don't know
DISTINGUISHING FEATURE: Very emotional
WHAT CAN'T YOU LIVE WITHOUT: Laughter,
dancing, creating, singing, loving
WHAT DO YOU DO AS A SPECIAL TREAT FOR
YOURSELF: Take the time to appreciate things
YOUR THREE SIGNATURE WARDROBE PIECES:
A black vinyl Wanda Nylon trench coat, a vintage
Yves Saint Laurent tuxedo, a vintage lamé dress
THREE MUST-HAVE BEAUTY PRODUCTS:
Sisley's Moisturizer with Cucumber, Yves Saint
Laurent's Touche Éclat (I don't go out without
it), and Benefit's Benetint cheek and lip stain
YOUR PERFUME: Memo's Shams Oud
WHO IS YOUR IDOL: I have none, since
the very definition of the word makes me
uncomfortable. I am more inspired by
people I know, by people close to me.
WHAT BOOK IS ON YOUR NIGHTSTAND:
Céline's *Journey to the End of Night*
YOUR LUCKY CHARM: I'm not superstitious
LESS OR MORE: More, obviously! Less is boring.
YOUR MOTTO: "Free the nipples!"
YOUR ADVICE FOR READERS:
Beauty is about personality.

Do you have a real walk-in closet? Yes, how lucky! At home, my partner and I share an entire room. It's a real dream: the walls are covered in tan leather and the doors are mirrored.
Is your closet orderly? Not really. I don't have the time for that. In any case I'm in such a hurry in the morning that I immediately make a big mess of it.
Should one keep accumulating clothes or regularly sort them out to keep only what is essential? I sort them regularly, otherwise there's just stuff everywhere.
What are the key items in your closet? The basics you can slip on in the morning without thinking. Lately, I'm in a jumpsuit phase. I design them and wear them all the time. You slip into it, and that's that. No need to think of what to wear with it. You can wear flats with it all day, and, in the evening, just put on some lipstick and the high heels hidden under your desk.
Do you have any UFOs in your closet? Tons. I'm rather adventurous.
New or vintage? Vintage, no question.
Cheap or chic? Cheap and chic! That's the trick.
Who tells the truth: the mirror or other people? I tell the truth, when I see myself, and depending on my mood and state of fatigue. It doesn't matter much what other people think.

DAY

06

PERFECTING MY

Skin

MY FOOLPROOF DAILY ROUTINE

SECRETS FOR A MAGNIFICENT COMPLEXION

"There is no finer, richer, more beautiful fabric than a beautiful woman's skin."

Anatole France

I
n this chapter we will discuss one of the most sensitive issues: THE SKIN.

Skin issues often come up in conversations with friends from the time we are teenagers with acne problems to a few years later when we yearn for fresh air and rest after parties or exhausting days of work. The worst of these skin crises has to be the topic of wrinkles and signs of aging.

Believe me, even models obsess over these things; you'd be surprised by how many of them do not have the gorgeous complexion you see on magazine covers.

And such concerns are far from frivolous; in fact they are perfectly legit when you consider that the skin, in terms of surface area, is our body's largest organ.

The skin is also linked to touch and thus to our sensitivity: it's our shield, protecting us from the outside world, receiving the softest caresses but also subjected to external aggression, such as harmful sun rays, cold weather, or injuries. This protective armor of ours, this envelope that represents us, requires tender loving care.

You'd never dream of starting the day without brushing your teeth or taking a shower, would you? Same goes for washing your face: you have to cleanse your skin. Often we don't become aware that our skin requires special treatment until our first wrinkles show up—and that's a mistake. The skin has a memory; it's a real resource that has to be taken care of every single day.

MY DAILY ROUTINE

DON'T WORRY,
THE SECRET TO GORGEOUS
SKIN IS WITHIN REACH AND
IS BASED ON ONE GOLDEN
RULE: A REGULAR SKINCARE
ROUTINE.

NARS Skin

gentle cream cleanser
crème nettoyante tout douceur

4.

shu uemura
TSUYA skin
youthful crystal-transparency lotion
lotion éclat cristal jeunesse

II

2.

3.

BOOSTER ANTI-AGE
INTERVENTION
RAPIDE

la prairie
SWITZERLAND

6.

la prairie

5.

CELLULAR
EYE MAKEUP
REMOVER
DÉMAQUILLANT
CELLULAIRE
POUR LES YEUX

la prairie
SWITZERLAND

1.

LA ROCHE-POSAY
LABORATOIRE DERMATOLOGIQUE

REDERMIC R
CORRECTEUR DERMATOLOGIQUE ANTI-ÂGE
ANTI-AGEING CONCENTRATE INTENSIVE

7.

HOW TO IDENTIFY
YOUR **SKIN TYPE**

NORMAL SKIN

My complexion is even and there are no apparent imperfections or signs of discomfort. It is luminous.

Facing page:

1. La Prairie, Cellular Eye Make-Up Remover
2. Shu Uemura, Tsuya Skin Youthful Crystal Transparency Lotion
3. Sensai, Cellular Performance Hydrachange Mask
4. Nars, Gentle Cream Cleanser
5. La Prairie, Anti-Aging Stress Cream
6. La Prairie, Anti-Aging Rapid Response Booster
7. La Roche-Posay, Redermic R: *anti-aging concentrate intensive*

SENSITIVE AND **DRY** SKIN

My skin isn't very soft, has red spots, is very thin, reactive, and prone to blotches and allergies, and does not defend itself well against aggressive external factors.

Right:

1. Crème de la Mer
2. Christian Dior, Capture Totale Dreamskin: *global age-defying skincare*
3. Shiseido, Perfect Cleansing Oil
4. La Prairie, Cellular Softening and Balancing Lotion
5. Dr. Brandt, Xtend Your Youth: *lip filler and volumizer*
6. Kiehl's, Super Multi-Corrective Eye-Opening Serum

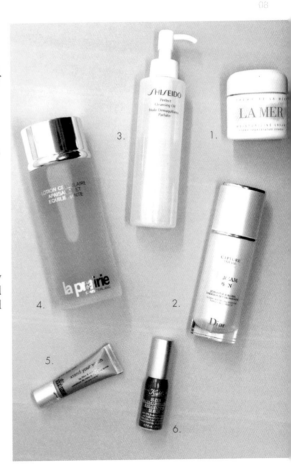

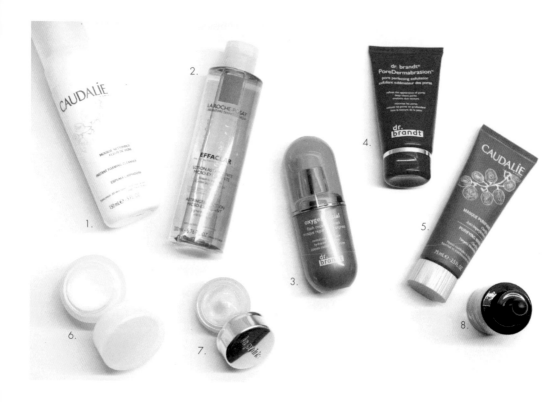

COMBINATION AND OILY SKIN

My skin is not even. It has normal, drier, and oilier zones, notably at the T-zone (forehead-nose-chin). Oily skin is thick and shiny, with dilated pores.

Above:

1. Caudalie, Instant Foaming Cleanser
2. La Roche-Posay, Effaclar Lotion:
   effaclar micro-exfoliating lotion
3. Dr. Brandt, Oxygen Facial: *flash recovery mask*
4. Dr. Brandt, PoreDermabrasion: *pore perfecting exfoliator*
5. Caudalie, Purifying Mask
6. Shiseido, Pureness Moisturizing Gel-Cream
7. La Prairie, Cellular Revitalizing Eye Gel
8. Caudalie, Overnight Detox Oil

MATURE SKIN

I am over fifty, and whether my skin is dry, normal, combination, or oily, it requires extra care.

Facing page:

1. La Prairie, Cellular Radiance Perfection Fluide Pure Gold
2. Kiehl's, Powerful Wrinkle Reducing Cream
3. Yves Saint Laurent, Or Rouge Eye Cream
4. Christian Dior, Diorific: *long-wearing lipstick*
5. Shu Uemura, Ultime8: *sublime beauty cleansing oil*
6. Shiseido, Benefiance NutriPerfect: *pro-fortifying softener*
7. Caudalie, Parfum Divin

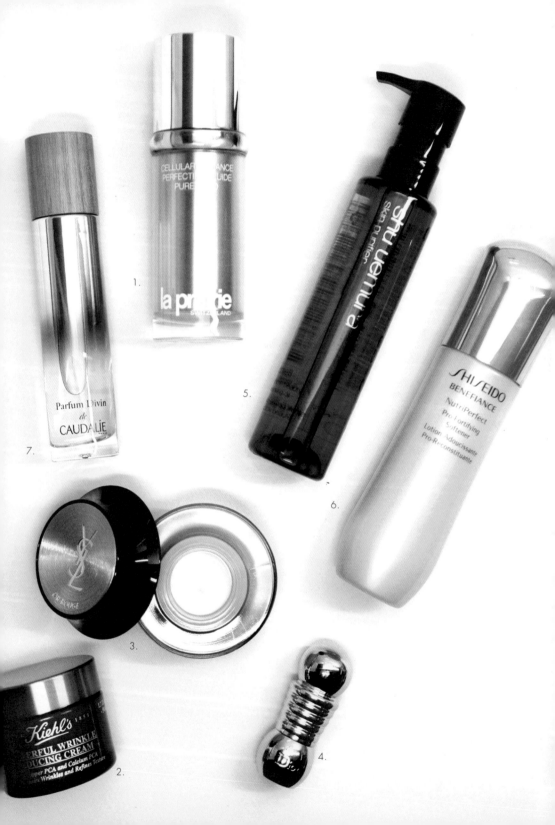

1. CELLULAR RADIANCE PERFECTING FLUIDE PURE GOLD
la prairie SWITZERLAND

2. Kiehl's 1851 POWERFUL WRINKLE REDUCING CREAM Super PCA and Calcium PCA Reduces Wrinkles and Refines Texture

3. YSL OR ROUGE

4. Dior

5. shu uemura skin purifier

6. SHISEIDO BENEFIANCE NutriPerfect Pro-Fortifying Softener Lotion Adoucissante Pro-Reconstituante

7. Parfum Divin de CAUDALIE

THE **ESSENTIAL** STEPS

The secret to fresh, luminous skin comes down to three simple steps:

- CLEANSE
- TONE
- HYDRATE

Be careful, however. We're not all the same when it comes to skin quality, and the creams and lotions the skin requires vary from one skin type to another.

1 **CLEANSE** YOUR SKIN

So many things can cause the skin to clog up: pollution, dust, sweat, traces of makeup, and bacteria. Our skin amasses all these elements, which aren't necessarily visible to the naked eye, and which lead to a loss of luminosity, so our skin looks dull.

It's important to cleanse the skin MORNING and EVENING. I myself am very lazy about doing it twice a day, but you'll be surprised by how much benefit you'll derive from being disciplined about it.

By cleansing your skin correctly, it will breathe better and be softer, firmer, and more luminous. A wide array of products of various textures exist—milks, oils, foams, and gels—to help purify your skin whatever its type. It's up to you to select whichever product is best for you.

I would be remiss if I didn't mention those handy little makeup remover wipes. While they are particularly well suited to our busy lifestyle, they must be used only occasionally. Obviously using a wipe is preferable to not removing your makeup at all if you come in late one night, or if you are not at your place and you want to change your makeup. But please be aware that wipes don't cleanse in depth. They always leave traces on your skin and do not replace a real makeup remover.

2 **TONE** YOUR SKIN

To be quite frank, it took me a long time to grasp what toners were really for. I thought you could skip this step. But since I've started using them in my daily routine, I can guarantee that not only do I get it, but I also understand how effective they are.

Toners are the ideal complement to in-depth cleansing. Toning completes the process of eliminating traces of makeup, restores your pH balance, and revitalizes and prepares the skin so that the creams and lotions you use next will penetrate more effectively.

These two steps can be pretty tedious and doing them on a daily basis requires real discipline. However, without them, there's no point in using any cream on your skin, no matter how expensive the product might be.

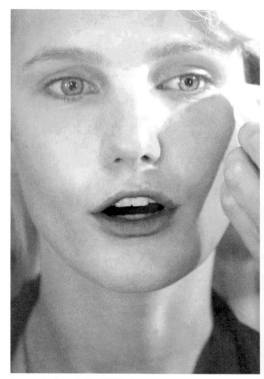

Anmari Botha - IMG MODELS.

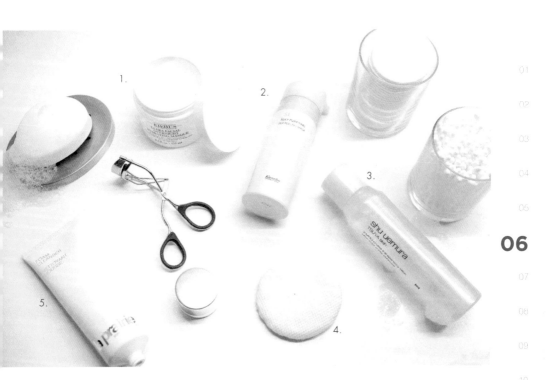

3 HYDRATE YOUR SKIN
As with cleansers, the range of hydrating products with innovative, varied textures is quite wide.

The best weapon for keeping wrinkles at bay is moisturizer. Moisturizing creams capture the water that makes up two-thirds of our skin and preserves just the right moisture level to prevent dehydration. Moisturizers create a protective barrier against little daily attacks.

Properly hydrated skin stays younger and suppler for a longer time. Ideally, apply your cream morning and evening and always keep in mind that hydrating your skin starts from the inside: drink plenty of water every day (1 ½ quarts [1.5 liters] minimum).

4 EXFOLIATE WITH A SCRUB
This is the ideal weekly complement to your daily routine. The aim of scrubbing is to remove the dead cells that make your epidermis look dull. What are its real benefits? Your skin will be:
- More luminous
- Visibly softer
- Less prone to wrinkles and fine lines
- Prepared to absorb all the treatments you will apply afterwards

Above:

1. Kiehl's, Ultra Facial Overnight Hydrating Mask
2. Sensai, Silk Peeling Mask
3. Shu Uemura, Tsuya Skin Youthful Crystal Transparency Lotion
4. Shiseido, Bio-Performance: super exfoliating disc
5. La Prairie, Foam Cleanser

IN ADDITION

5 MICRODERMABRASION

Up until about ten years ago, micro-dermabrasion was carried out in beauty salons, only. Dr. Brandt was among the first to introduce the ritual to home users. It is sort of an in-depth super-scrub. It helps eliminate spots, scars, traces of acne, wrinkles, and fine lines. It involves applying an abrasive product made up of aluminum oxide micro-crystals. However, if your skin is very sensitive, dry, or acne-prone, the technique must be avoided. It is also contraindicated for pregnant women. Following treatment, using cream with a high SPF is recommended to hydrate and protect the skin and to keep spots from appearing. You should also avoid exposure to the sun for three days following the treatment.

ESSENTIAL PRODUCTS

1 ANTIOXIDANTS

Antioxidants are products that help us combat free radicals and pollution, which are responsible for premature skin aging.

Our skin naturally contains antioxidants, but we can increase their level by seeking out foods naturally rich in them. For example, apples contain retinol, which triggers the production of collagen and vitamin C, which itself improves the skin's luminosity.

2 SERUMS AND MASKS

Serums and masks strengthen and boost the effect of your daily skin treatments.

Why use a serum? Contrary to creams that only penetrate the superficial layers of the epidermis, serums act more in-depth due to their gel textures with a higher concentration of active ingredients. A serum is your daily skincare product's best friend.

Why use a mask? Masks intensify your treatment's targeted action. They are a kind of weekly reward for your skin. More intimate than the daily routine, they are like a romantic night in with your skin: one evening a week in a quiet place, after a good bath, apply a mask, like a magic ritual.

3 EYE CONTOUR CREAMS AND LIP BALMS

The eye contours and lips are the most sensitive areas of the face, where the skin is finer and the first signs of aging appear. Yet these two zones are the very ones we frequently forget to hydrate and repair. They require targeted treatment.

You mustn't wait for your first wrinkles to show up before you start to deal with them.

The eye contours: though gels have an antifatigue effect and are recommended when you have under-eye puffiness, creams deal more specifically with fine lines, while other products minimize dark circles.

Lip balms offer wrinkle treatment for the upper lip to prevent chapping and dryness, and are your everyday allies.

THE ENEMIES OF RADIANT SKIN

We all have a genetic heritage that we cannot change. Taking care of our skin with a daily routine is the best way of sustaining it.

However, beyond the routine and the skin treatments, we must also be aware that our lifestyle has a huge influence on our complexion, both positively and negatively. Below are the factors that you must absolutely master if you want to maintain a healthy complexion and firm skin:

- SUN
- SMOKING
- DRINKING
- LACK OF SLEEP
- POLLUTION

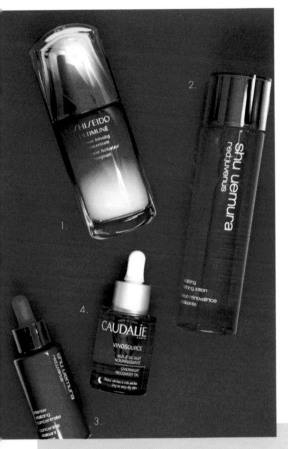

Left:
1. Shiseido, Power Infusing Concentrate
2. Shu Uemura, Red:Juvenus: *revitalizing refining lotion*
3. Shu Uemura, Red:Juvenus: *intense vitalizing concentrate*
4. Caudalie, Vinosource: *overnight recovery oil*

FOR **PERFECT SKIN**

EVERY DAY
- I cleanse my skin, morning and evening
- I use my **toner**
- I apply my **moisturizing cream**

ONCE A WEEK
- I **exfoliate** with a scrub
- I apply a **moisturizing mask**

WHAT ARE YOUR FAVORITE SKINCARE PRODUCTS?
\# #getgorgeous, #beautychallenge21

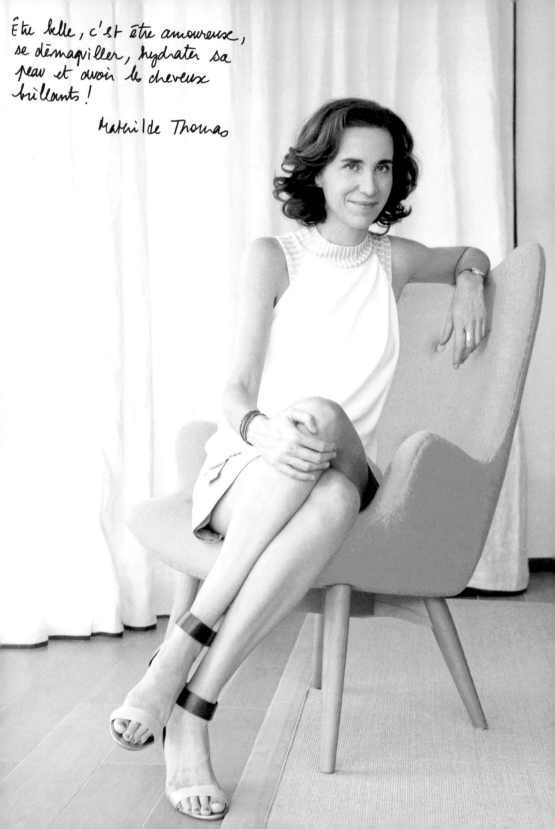

Être belle, c'est être amoureuse,
se démaquiller, hydrater sa
peau et avoir les cheveux
brillants !

Mathilde Thomas

Mathilde Thomas

AGE: 44
PROFESSION: Caudalie cofounder
FIRST JOB: Internship in a wonderful perfume house in Grasse, France
YOUR FAVORITE PHOTO OF YOURSELF: A black-and-white picture my father took of me pouting at age seven
ASTROLOGICAL SIGN: Sagittarius
DISTINGUISHING FEATURE: 5'8" (1m60)
WHAT CAN'T YOU LIVE WITHOUT: Love
WHAT DO YOU DO AS A SPECIAL TREAT FOR YOURSELF: I get a massage
YOUR THREE SIGNATURE WARDROBE PIECES: Jeans, white shirt, sneakers
THREE MUST-HAVE BEAUTY PRODUCTS: Premier Cru The Cream, Beauty Elixir, Divine Oil; all from Caudalie, of course
YOUR PERFUME: Caudalie's Thé des Vignes
WHO IS YOUR IDOL: My grandmother
WHAT BOOK IS ON YOUR NIGHTSTAND: Patrick Suskind's *Perfume*
YOUR LUCKY CHARM: An old silver flask pendant, from Hermès
LESS OR MORE: Less
YOUR MOTTO: "They did not know it was impossible, so they did it." —Mark Twain
YOUR ADVICE FOR READERS: Carefully remove your makeup morning and evening. Moisturize your skin, protect it from the sun, and do a scrub and mask twice a week.

What is your skin type? Combination.
What are your secrets for pampering skin that shows signs of sleep deprivation?
I start the day with a detox mask, I moisturize abundantly, then I use lots of tinted cream, bronzing powder, and a dark circle concealer.
What would your beauty prescription be?
A good, 100% natural makeup remover oil, an antioxidant moisturizing cream, SPF 50 sunscreen cream, tinted cream, a good detox mask.
What are three quality, low-priced cosmetics products? At Caudalie, the Micellar Cleansing Water, the Moisturizing Sorbet, the Instant Detox Mask.
Are you a fan of organic cosmetics? Organics are better than before but we aren't yet there in terms of effectiveness, scent, and cosmetics quality.

———

Facing page: To be beautiful is to be in love, wash your face, moisturize your skin, and have shiny hair.

DAY

07

MASTERING MY

Hair

EVERY DAY IS A GOOD HAIR DAY

WE ALL WANT MORE **BEAUTIFUL, HEALTHY,** AND **MANAGEABLE** HAIR

"Beauty in the skies lies in the stars;
beauty in women lies in their hair."

Italian proverb

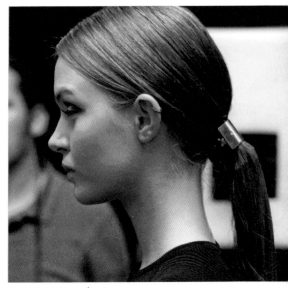

Josephine Skriver - Élite Paris.

T he expression "I want to tear my hair out" can certainly resonate when you catch a glimpse of yourself in the mirror in the morning.

Say goodbye to that fantastic blow-dry you got at the hairdresser's and hello to the humongous cowlick your pillow provided. If you've had your color done as well, hello to roots.

That panicky feeling you get looking in the bathroom mirror is a classic, much like the alarm bells that ring when you stare into your closet (*see* Day 5). To avoid this nightmare so you can do your hair quickly (*see* Day 9), you have to follow a few rules.

75

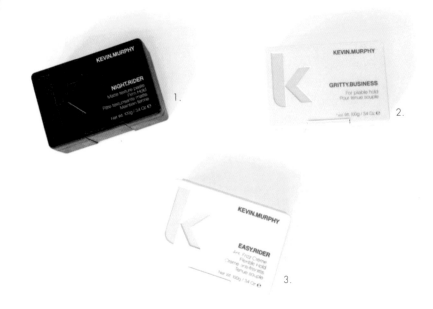

From Kevin.Murphy (above):
1. Night.Rider, Matte Texture Paste: *firm hold*

2. Gritty.Business: *pliable hold*
3. Easy.Rider, Anti Frizz Crème: *flexible hold*

1 Don't wash your hair every day. The scalp naturally produces sebum—the secretion that makes your hair shine and whose purpose is to protect it. The more you wash your hair, the more you spur the sebaceous glands to produce a lipidic film and the more quickly the hair seems to become dirty. It's a vicious circle.

If you aren't able to space out your shampoos, the alternative is to do a dry shampoo, which works very well. You'll find products for all hair colors at Bumble & Bumble.

2 Brush your hair before you wash it. This way you'll keep it from getting too tangled as you wash it. Use a brush with natural fibers. The Mason Pearson boar-bristle and nylon brushes are a real reference. By brushing, you spread the sebum out over your hair, so it's better protected from shampoo.

3 Do your final rinse with cold water to close up the hair cuticle and make your hair shine.

4 To untangle wet hair, always use a wide-tooth comb. The Leonor Greyl comb is perfect. Fine combs break the hair fibers.

5 Leave on your product (shampoo, mask, and conditioner) for the time indicated. We are all pressed for time but this is essential. On a daily basis you can take advantage of the waiting time to wash your body. On the weekend, treat yourself to a special beauty moment for your hair, like you do for your face and body. Draw a bath in a calm setting, apply your mask, and wrap your hair in a warm towel to boost the effect of the treatment. You can even leave your mask on all night.

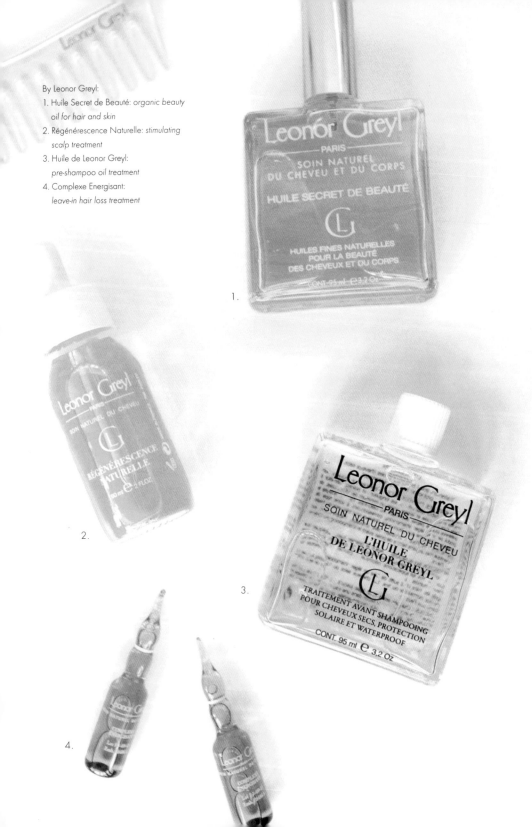

By Leonor Greyl:

1. Huile Secret de Beauté: *organic beauty oil for hair and skin*
2. Régénérescence Naturelle: *stimulating scalp treatment*
3. Huile de Leonor Greyl: *pre-shampoo oil treatment*
4. Complexe Energisant: *leave-in hair loss treatment*

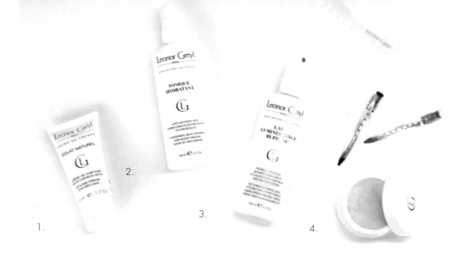

From Leonor Greyl (above):

1. Eclat Naturel: *nourishing and protecting styling cream*

2. Tonique Hydratant: *leave-in moisturizing mist*

3. Lait Luminescence: *leave-in detangling and protective spray*

4. Baume Bois de Rose: *modelling and sculpting balm - matte finish*

6 Dry your hair in a towel as gently as if you were patting your face dry. Twisting and rubbing the hair too roughly will break the fibers and open the hair cuticles, inviting frizziness.

7 Use hair oil treatments. The night before your shampoo, spray your hair with oil (there are very good ones at Leonor Greyl and Caudalie), brush it to spread the product to the ends of the hair and let the oil set until the next day. This is an excellent routine for dry, curly, frizzy, and colored hair.

8 My dad always said, "There are no good workers without good tools." The quality of the products you use is important, but the quality of your brushes, combs, hair bands, and pins is every bit as significant. Even if they cost more, combs made of horn and brushes of boar bristle are an excellent investment.

9 Be careful not to use hair bands or pins in wet hair: the hair fibers shrink while drying and could break.

10 Use flat irons and blow-dryers in moderation. Never use them at maximum temperature. Flat irons should never be used at more than 350°F/180°C. Targeted products exist to help you protect your hair from aggressive heat, as needed.

11 Be wary of fixative products containing alcohol, like strong hairspray or gels, which dehydrate your hair. A better option is a gentler type of finishing product like wax or serum, whose suppler texture protects and hydrates hair fibers rather than mistreating them.

12 In the same way that you protect your skin from the sun, think about protecting your hair in summer. Use sunscreens, use masks more frequently, and, above all, rinse out your hair after swimming in saltwater or chlorinated water.

13 Cut your hair approximately once every two months, even if only a quarter of an inch. This keeps split ends from doing real damage to your hair, and will improve your hair's overall health.

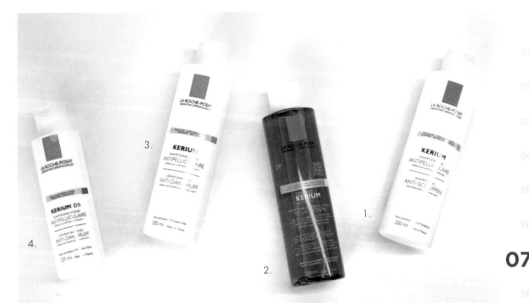

DANDRUFF

This problem affects a lot of us. Dandruff flakes form on the scalp and cause redness; they can provoke itching, and then make an unsightly appearance on your shoulders. Dandruff can be genetic, but stress is a major factor in making it worse.

The right treatment depends on whether you have oily or dry dandruff flakes:

- Oily dandruff: **Kerium Anti-Dandruff Gel-Shampoo** (1) from La Roche-Posay; their no-rinse, botanical tonic is also well suited to the problem.

- Dry dandruff: **Kerium Anti-Dandruff Cream-Shampoo** (3) from La Roche-Posay.

- Persistent dandruff: **Kerium DS Anti-Dandruff Intensive Shampoo** (4) from La Roche-Posay.

Because an ounce of prevention is worth a pound of cure, we recommend you use essential oils such as Leonor Greyl's **Régénérescence Naturelle** oil (see p. 77, number 2), which purifies and stimulates the scalp while preventing dandruff.

From La Roche-Posay, Kerium range (above):
1. Oily Dandruff: *anti-dandruff gel shampoo*
2. Extra Gentle Physiological Gel-Shampoo with La Roche-Posay thermal spring water
3. Dry Dandruff: *anti-dandruff cream shampoo*
4. DS Anti-Dandruff Intensive Micro Exfoliating Treatment Shampoo

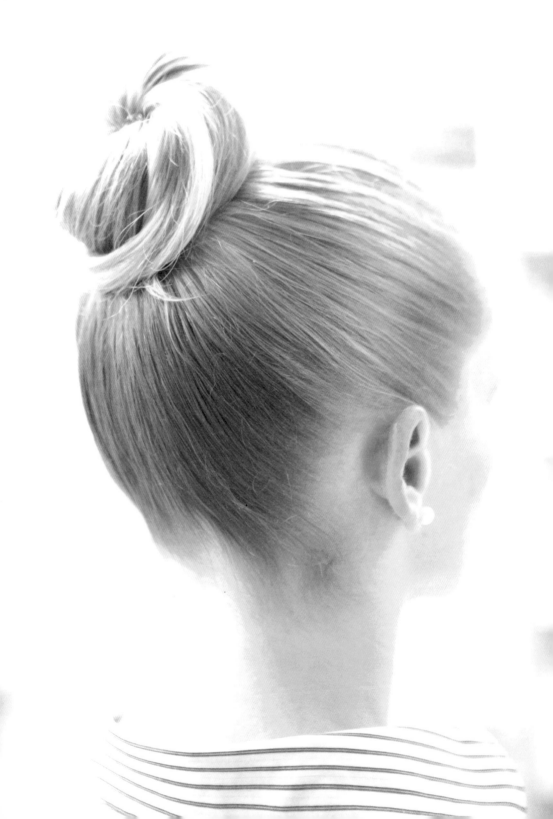

TYPES OF **HAIR**

FINE HAIR

Fine hair is brittler than normal hair. It is important not to use oily products on this kind of hair. They will only weigh it down even more. Use special products for dry hair, like Leonor Greyl's **Shampooing au Miel**, or Paul Mitchell's **Extra-Body** line. Having fine hair myself, my hairdresser has always told me to get a layered cut, which reduces the weight of the hair and gives it volume and shape. For the same reasons, you shouldn't wear your hair too long if it is fine. Shoulder length at maximum. Another trick is never to use conditioner on the roots, only on the ends of your hair, and always dry your hair with your head upside down. Finally, there are styling foams that boost the volume of your hair, like Leonor Greyl's **Mousse au Lotus Volumatrice**.

OILY HAIR

Don't worry: oily hair is a common problem.

Oiliness is due to over-secretion of sebum, so it's important to use the right shampoo.

For those with hair that is oily at the roots but drier (or colored) at the ends, we recommend the Kérastase shampoo **Bain Divalent**.

Absolutely avoid touching your hair during the day. Do not brush it except when you go to wash it. This will keep from overly stimulating the sebaceous glands.

A tip from my hairdresser: wash your brushes, combs, and accessories once a week in warm water and disinfect them with iso-propryl alcohol (91%).

Remember, heat stimulates sebum secre-tion: it's important to avoid using hot water when washing your hair and to keep your blow-dryer heat to a minimum as well.

DRY OR FRIZZY HAIR

Why does hair become dry and devitalized? Dry hair is hair that has lost its protective film and consequently has become dehydrated. It becomes brittler and tends to break or frizz. To prevent the effects of dehydration, it's important to space out shampoos to a maximum. Oils are great allies, helping to reestablish your hair's natural protection system. The Leonor Greyl oils are perfect for that. Caudalie's are very good, also. Apply oil one or two hours prior to shampooing your hair or, better, leave it on all night. Avoid washing your hair with overly warm water, which makes it brittle; lukewarm water is ideal. Be careful to use shampoos and masks suited to your hair type. For dry or frizzy hair, we recommend the Sebastian shampoo and mask **Penetraitt** and **Potion 9** respectively, which restore hair fibers in depth. Use a warm towel to enhance their effects. It is very important to avoid using a blow-dryer, curling irons, and ceramic plate irons. Allowing your hair to dry naturally is ideal, but if the resulting texture does not suit you (if your hair is too fluffy), try products like Leonor Greyl's **Éclat Naturel** cream or **Sérum de Soie Sublimateur**.

Should you want to use one of these kinds of heated appliances, use thermo-protective products to minimize the damage caused by heat on the hair fibers.

Our favorite trick: Redken's **Anti-Snap** that prevents breakage.

COLORED OR HIGHLIGHTED HAIR

My first piece of advice if you have colored or highlighted hair is: do not do it yourself. Rely on good professionals so you'll get flawless results. Doing this kind of technical operation at home increases the risk of damaging your hair. Coloring the hair (highlights, California highlights, bleach) is a very tricky process that, to be honest, is quite aggressive: it's essential for a qualified professional to do the job.

My tip: avoid washing your hair the day before having it colored.

To increase the amount of time your color and shine will last, follow the advice below:

Use special products for colored hair (shampoos and masks), which will both nourish the hair and preserve its color.

Remember that colored hair is more porous and sensitive. In summer, protect it with the right products to prevent color-altering aggression from the outside (pool, sun, seawater).

Our prescription: Redkin's **Color Extend** line and Leonor Greyl's **Bain Vitalisant B** shampoo **Crème Régénératrice** conditioner.

HAIR LOSS

Very fortunately women are genetically less prone than men to hair loss. However, stress, the use of aggressive products, and a poor diet can make the phenomenon worse. If you suffer from significant hair loss, avoid coffee and smoking.

Helpful hints to salvage the situation:

- Every day lightly **massage your scalp** to help slow hair loss while improving the blood supply.
- At all costs **avoid** using overly **tight hair bands**.
- Keep your **blow-dryer** at least a foot from your head and use it at **low temperature**.

If these tricks are not enough, you can also do an intensive treatment with food supplements, such as René Furterer's **Vitalfan** gelcaps, or use energizing ampoules such as Leonor Greyl's **Complexe Énergisant**, which you apply by micromassaging and allowing the product to penetrate into the scalp.

POST A PHOTO OF YOUR FAVORITE HAIRSTYLE.
#getgorgeous, #beautychallenge21

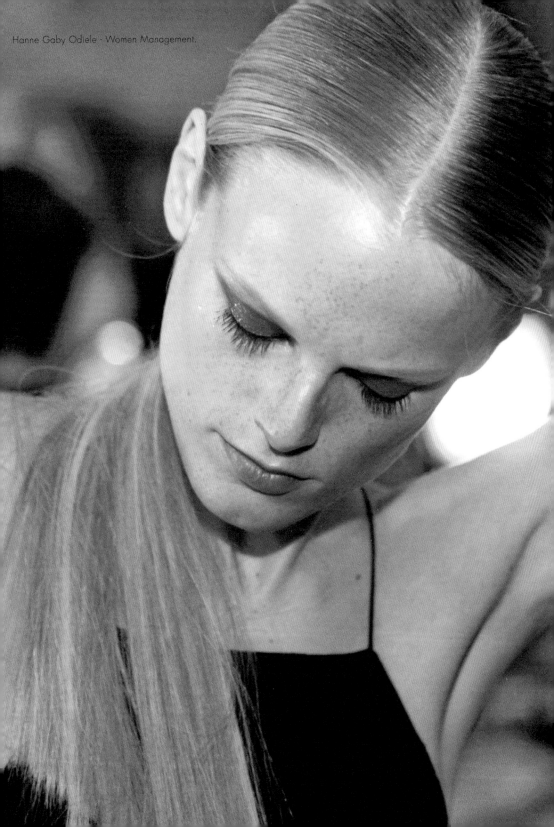

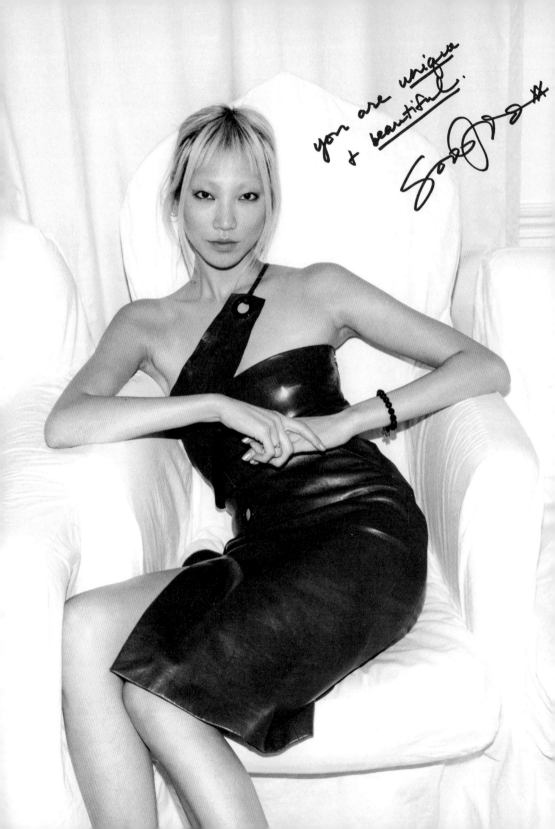

you are unique
+ beautiful.

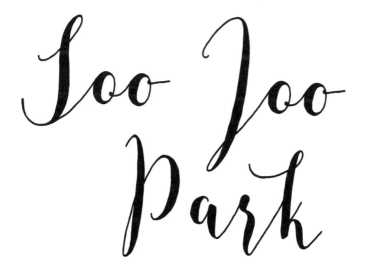

Soo Joo Park

AGE: 29
PROFESSION: Model
FIRST JOB: Librarian at my college library, shelving books
ASTROLOGICAL SIGN: Aries
DISTINGUISHING FEATURE: Bleached hair and a sharp jawline
WHAT CAN'T YOU LIVE WITHOUT: Love and my iPhone
WHAT DO YOU DO AS A SPECIAL TREAT FOR YOURSELF: After long trips, I always go to a spa for a massage and a scrub
YOUR THREE SIGNATURE WARDROBE PIECES: Shredded jeans, Chelsea boots, a silver necklace with a tassel charm
THREE MUST-HAVE BEAUTY PRODUCTS: Officinali di Montauto's OM Skincare Baume Viso Tonic, L'Oréal Paris Colour Riche Lipstick in Beige A Nu 630, Tom Ford Shade & Illuminate highlighter and shader duo
YOUR PERFUME: Chanel No. 5
WHO IS YOUR IDOL: David Bowie
WHAT BOOK IS ON YOUR NIGHTSTAND: *A Season In Hell* and *The Drunken Boat* by Arthur Rimbaud; *Birthday Stories* by Haruki Murakami
LESS OR MORE? Less
YOUR MOTTO: "You Only Live Once (YOLO)."
YOUR ADVICE FOR READERS: Don't let others define you.

What is your hair like naturally? Silky, straight black hair.

Short or long? Natural or dyed? Long and platinum! I wish I was naturally a bleach blonde!

What was your worst hair moment? The hair around my crown broke off a couple of times due to severe damage and bleach overlapping while I was touching up my roots. I wore a lot of hats and learned a lot of tricks from that.

What's the best advice a hairdresser ever gave you? Before a visit to bleach your roots, apply lots of coconut oil to your scalp for protection.

What hair care tips do you recommend? Take supplements like biotin (vitamin B8) regularly and stop picking at the ends—it causes more damage.

Your favorite hair products? Redken Extreme Length Sealer split-end treatment, Milbon Noiraudepro reconstructive hair treatment, coconut oil, the Redken Blonde Idol BBB Spray Multi-Benefit Hair Treatment.

How do you protect your hair from heat damage and dryness during the summer? I try to avoid using any heating devices and request that stylists use the lowest heat setting during shoots and shows. I apply a lot of oil and serums like coconut oil and Redken Extreme Length Sealer. Twice a week I do at-home hair treatments using Redken Extreme Strength Builder Plus Hair Mask.

DAY

08

TAKING CARE OF MY

Body

MY DAILY RITUALS

YOUR **BODY** IS WHERE YOU **LIVE**

"We are what we repeatedly do. Excellence, then, is not an action, but a habit."

Aristotle

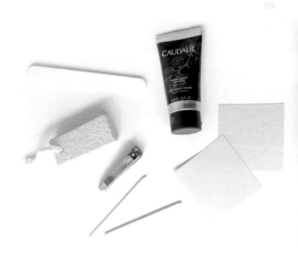

Caudalie, Foot Beauty Cream.

Taking care of your body is, above all, a way of loving yourself and others, since it's through the body that you present yourself to the world. Gracefulness, attractiveness, and elegance come from your body and how you inhabit it. Holding yourself well, having good posture and graceful gestures, is quite an art, which has nothing to do with weight or shape.

Slenderness is not everything: I am aware of the impact and influence fashion photos have on women. It's true that the fashion world values slenderness, even skinniness. It's complex. From a purely aesthetic perspective, I appreciate slenderness in models, since it really highlights the clothes. But I know the power of images, the impact of the dictate of slenderness, and the traumatic reactions images can cause, particularly in young women.

So to all those who may have become depressed on seeing a special "weight loss"

issue of a magazine, I would like to reassure you: models are not perfect, either, and thinness does not make a body more desirable.

So keep in mind that thinness is not the ultimate goal: above all, being gorgeous means being at peace with your body.

As you can see, this book is first and foremost a guide to self-love.

Life is made up of change, and a woman's life is constantly evolving. There are three major acts, which Jane Fonda explains so well in her book *Prime Time* (Random House, 2011): "In attempting to chart a course for myself into my sixties and beyond, I've found it helpful to view the symphony of my own life in three acts, or three major developmental stages: Act I, the first three decades; Act II, the middle three decades; and Act III, the final three decades (or however many more years one is granted)."

From adolescence to old age, our body undergoes significant hormonal changes. At every stage we must provide it with proper care and attention. After all we live in our body our entire life. Whether you are a young girl, woman, mother, or mature woman, the ball is now in your court.

Our body expresses what we are: our joy and pain, both past or present. Our physical condition often reflects the attention we give it. **So above all, love yourself!**

IMPORTANT APPOINTMENTS

These steps to maintain health and daily hygiene also help make us attractive! Don't neglect the relevant medical exams that correspond to your age:

- ❑ Gynecologist
- ❑ Dentist
- ❑ Podiatrist/Pedicure
- ❑ Osteopath
- ❑ Physical therapist

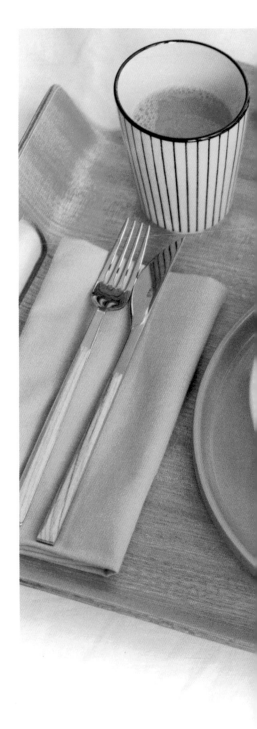

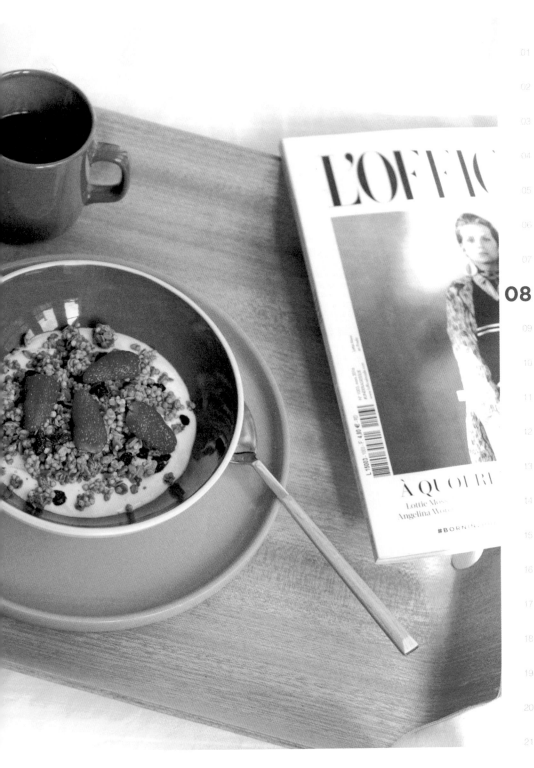

TAKING CARE OF YOUR **BODY** IS THE BASIS OF **WELL-BEING**

Having goals, making projections, looking at yourself, and pampering yourself all take time, so I suggest you follow a three-phase plan: yearly, monthly, weekly.

Whatever your habits, it's never too late to do a good job.

The idea isn't to set unattainable goals but to do simple things that will make your life easier. It's about establishing beauty routines and a healthy lifestyle. No matter what's in our genes, we are all beautiful in our own way.

Though you may already know much of what I'm about to say, it's sometimes good to repeat certain obvious facts. So don't forget: beauty, above all, lies inside you!

YEARLY

DIET

I am careful about my diet and eat in a healthy, balanced way. I favor vegetables and fruit, food with little fat, and I avoid sugar and forego the snacking that many of us give into. Frugality is synonymous with longevity.

With detox fads now in fashion, it's preferable to eat less but better quality food.

SLEEP

I sleep like a baby! Sleep is essential for well-being:
- It's good for the eyesight.
- It strengthens the immune system.
- It reduces stress and anxiety.
- It improves memory and intellectual capacity.

EXERCISE

Moving around and getting oxygen is one of the keys to well-being.

When you exercise, the body releases hormones like endorphins and dopamine, with mood-enhancing powers. Regular exercise makes it possible to feel better and better and to set goals for yourself. Plus, it's such a joy to make progress. It's good for the heart and mind, so make a small effort, and you're off. You'll have no regrets. Feeling good is not that complicated, but it involves a fair amount of commitment. Pilates or postural gymnastics, yoga or muscle strengthening exercises are terrific allies if you persevere on a daily basis!

DIETARY TIPS

- Never completely fill your plate
- Never take a second helping
- Eat light meals in the evening

"WE MUST
EAT LIKE
A PRINCE IN
THE MORNING,
A MERCHANT AT
NOON, AND
A POOR PERSON
AT NIGHT."

CHINESE PROVERB

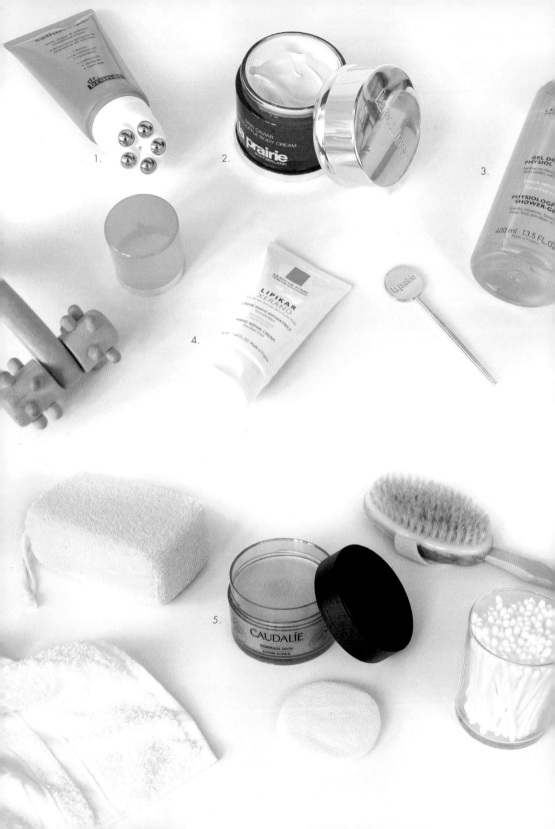

MONTHLY

DEPILATION
Depending on how much body hair you have, try different techniques to find the right one for you. Today there are many solutions that exist, but it's best to go to a beauty institute. The job is always better done by a professional.

For those who prefer doing it themselves: choose between shaving, waxing, electric shavers, hair removal cream, lasers, intense pulsed light—it's up to you to see what's best for you.

HAIRDRESSER
Getting your haircut and color done is key (*see* Day 7).

1. Dr. Brandt, Cellusculpt: *body shaper and cellulite smoothing cream*
2. La Prairie, Skin Caviar: *luxe soufflé body cream*
3. La Roche-Posay, Physiological Shower Gel
4. La Roche-Posay, Lipikar Xerand: *hand repair cream*

WEEKLY

Just like for the face (*see* Day 6), it's important to regularly do body scrubs, particularly when the seasons change. There are special products for this, such as those shown on the facing page. Or you can have a professional treatment done.

MANICURE
Having clean, elegant nails is crucial. For the bravest of us, there are very well-done kits that include the protective base, polish, and top coat. But again, there is always the professional salon, and fortunately there are more and more of them.

5. Caudalie, Divine Scrub
6. Chanel, Nail Colour Remover
7. Dior, Nail Glow
8. Dior, Vernis Wonderland 575

08

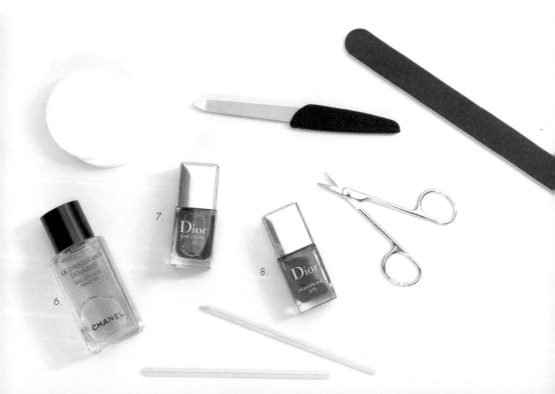

TIPS FOR A GOOD NIGHT'S SLEEP

Prepare your night like a day that's just starting:
- Air out your room, dab two or three drops of essential oil behind your ears.
- Take a hot shower or bath to relax!
- Stay away from screens that perk you up and instead read or meditate: a few minutes of quiet contemplation about the day you just spent will help you sleep well.
- Do a positive rundown of your day: what good things did you do? What could you do better tomorrow, without pressure? The idea is to see life from a positive angle. Be ZEN and POSITIVE!

EXERCISE TIPS

- Download yoga or Pilates-type apps on your Smartphone.
- Do 10 minutes of stretching exercises every morning.
- Climb the stairs and walk as much as possible.
- Dance!
- Buy a trampoline!

DAY
08
PAMPER MY BODY:
To-do list

1. FOOD

....
....
....
....

2. SLEEP

....
....
....
....

3. EXERCISE

....
....
....
....

4. OTHER

....
....
....
....

WHAT DID YOU DO TODAY TO CARE FOR YOUR BODY?
 # #getgorgeous, #beautychallenge21

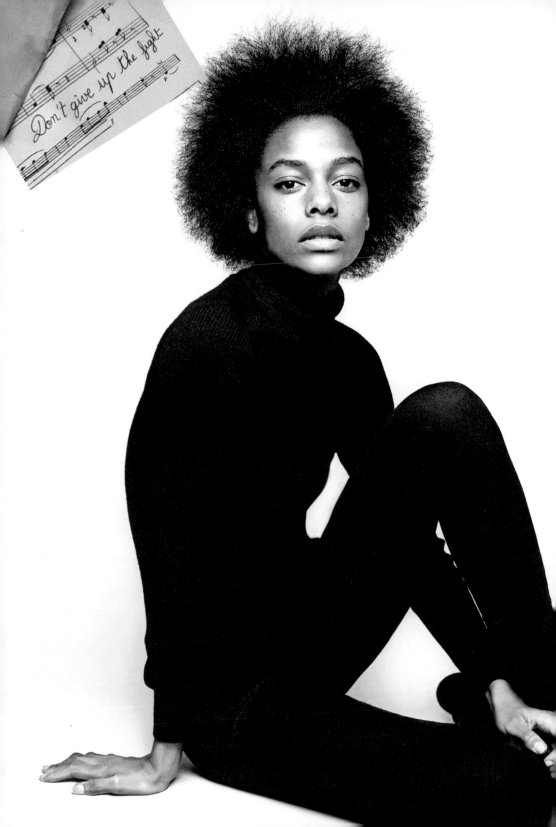

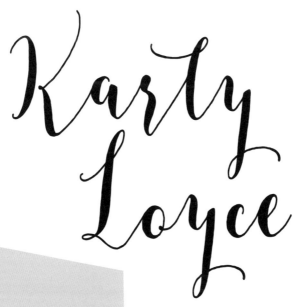

Karly Loyce

AGE: 23
PROFESSION: Model
YOUR FAVORITE PHOTO OF YOURSELF:
The one on the cover of *i-D* magazine, which
was my first shoot in New York. When I see it,
I realize how far I've come since that time.
ASTROLOGICAL SIGN: Libra
DISTINGUISHING FEATURE: The freckles on my face
WHAT CAN'T YOU LIVE WITHOUT: Music
WHAT DO YOU DO AS A SPECIAL TREAT FOR
YOURSELF: Spend time with people close
to me, go to the movies, go out to eat, or
go to the beach when I'm in Martinique
YOUR THREE SIGNATURE WARDROBE
PIECES: Jeans, shirts, and sneakers
THREE MUST-HAVE BEAUTY PRODUCTS:
Moisturizing creams for the face and body,
plant oils for my hair, makeup remover
YOUR PERFUME: Yves Saint Laurent's Black Opium
WHO IS YOUR IDOL: My mother
WHAT BOOK IS ON YOUR NIGHTSTAND:
The Little Prince by Antoine de Saint Exupéry
YOUR LUCKY CHARM: Every day is a lucky charm
LESS OR MORE: More: I love to fight for my dreams
YOUR MOTTO: "Never stop believing in
your dreams, and always persevere!"
YOUR ADVICE FOR READERS: Do all you can
to be happy and fulfilled; life is way too short
to allow stress and other daily problems to take over.
Think POSITIVE!

**Do you have to be thin to feel good about your
body?** NO! To feel good about your body, you
must, above all, accept yourself as you are.
How can you treat your body well? The
first thing is to like yourself. Then, keep
fit by eating right and exercising.
Your favorite part of your body: My legs.
Treatments: homemade or professional?
Homemade, especially for my hair care.
Your body-care prescription: For the shower,
use liquid soap (Ushuaia). After showering,
use a moisturizing cream with shea butter (Le
Petit Marseillais) to keep your skin moisturized
all day. Once a week, use an exfoliating liquid
soap to spur your cells to regenerate.
**What do you think of the way women's bodies are
represented in magazines?** It's often stereotyped:
thin, sexy, young, etc. But in reality we're all beautiful.
We just have to accept ourselves as we are. We're
all different: it would be good for magazines to
show this, so that readers could identify with
the models they present and not feel left out.

DAY

09

MASTERING 10-MINUTE

Makeup
AND
Hair

A LOOK THAT LASTS ALL DAY

PUT ON A LITTLE
MAKEUP

*"If you're unhappy,
put on some lipstick and attack!"*

Coco Chanel

Contrary to certain preconceived ideas, makeup is not pointless window dressing. Being well groomed and well made up is a symbol of femininity for women. How lucky we are to be able to embellish our features, to brighten up our face with color.

In previous chapters we learned how to take care of our skin, hair, and body, so now let's check out the key steps involved in having flawless all-day makeup along with a hairstyle that holds.

Everyone knows what it feels like to have an off day when you find yourself in a rotten mood because of unruly hair or because your makeup did not stay put.

As a teenager I was fascinated by 1950s pin-ups and more generally by the whole era when women wore elegant hats and had stylish hairdos and makeup.

I love that 1950s look and I adopted it when I turned fourteen. Today I still wear my makeup—red lipstick and black eyeliner—the same way. As certain models have told me, it's my signature.

Now it's your turn to identify or find your own signature look. Grab your makeup brushes!

MY **10-MINUTE** FLAWLESS **MAKEUP** ROUTINE

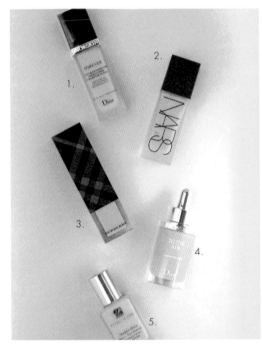

THE BASIC STEPS

Apply to well-cleansed and toned skin:

1. A serum: to boost the effect
   of the hydrating cream.
2. A base/hydrating cream: for soft,
   well-moisturized skin.
3. Foundation: to even the complexion
   and smooth the features.
4. A corrector and/or dark circle concealer:
   to erase signs of fatigue
   and provide light.
5. Loose and/or compact powder: to fix
   foundation and provide a matte finish.
6. An eyebrow pencil: to intensify eyes
   by accentuating the brow color.
7. Eye shadow: to brighten the eyes
   by creating contrast and depth.
8. Eye liner and/or pencil: to underline
   and widen the eyes.
9. Mascara: to give lashes thickness
   and length; it enhances the eyes.
10. Blush: for a healthy-glow.
11. Lip pencil: to reshape the lip contours
    and keep lipstick from smearing.
12. Lipstick: for the ultimate feminine touch.
13. Gloss: To give lips a beautiful shine.

This may seem painstaking, but in reality
these steps are easy to do. Try it
and you'll see it's worth the effort!

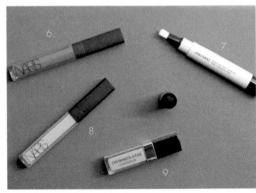

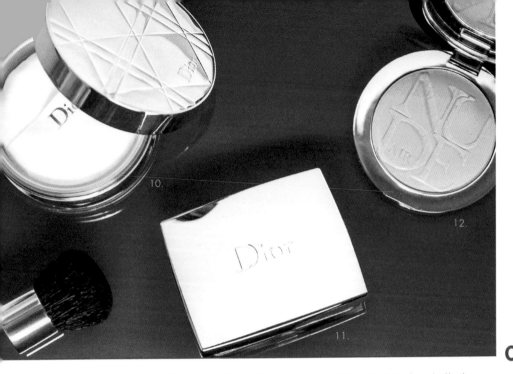

1. Dior, Diorskin Forever: *perfect makeup everlasting wear*
2. Nars, All Day Luminous Weightless Foundation
3. Burberry, Fresh Glow Luminous Fluid Base
4. Dior, Diorskin Nude Air Serum

5. Estée Lauder, Double Wear: *stay-in-place make-up*
6. Nars Cosmetics, Radiant Creamy Concealer
7. Shiseido, Sheer Eye Zone Corrector
8. Nars Cosmetics, Radiant Creamy Concealer
9. Dior, Diorskin Star Concealer

10. Dior, Diorskin Nude Air: *healthy glow invisible loose powder*
11. Dior, Eye Reviver: *illuminating neutrals eye palette*
12. Dior, Diorskin Nude Air: *healthy glow invisible powder*

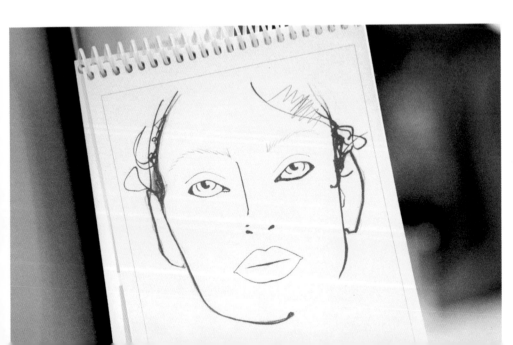

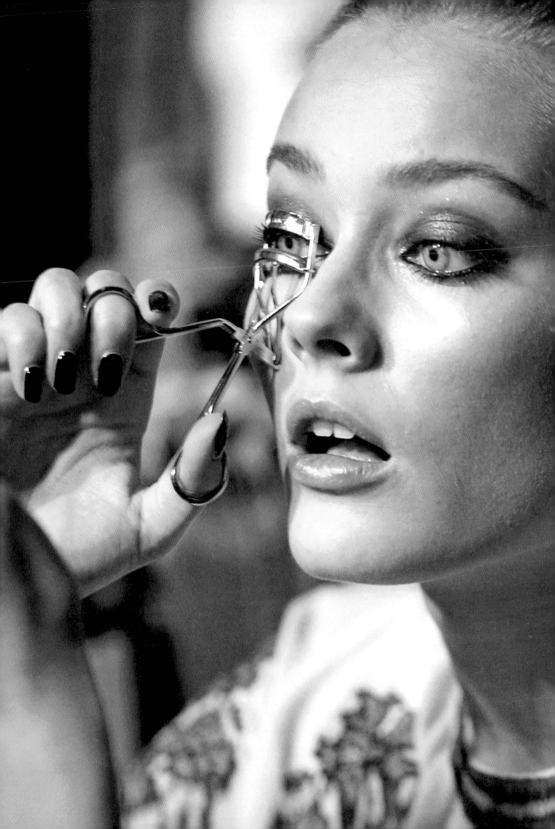

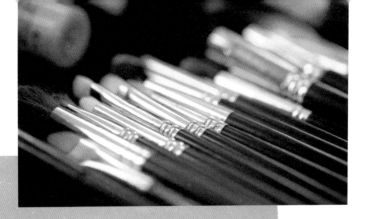

THE RIGHT **TOOLS** FOR
APPLYING MAKEUP

- Flat brushes/round ball brushes
- Big thick brushes, either round or flat:
  to apply foundation, powder, and blush –
  remember to wash them afterward
- Sponges and Beauty Blenders: for applying
  foundation or dark circle concealer
- Lash curlers: to curl lashes before
  putting on your mascara

IF YOU'RE NOT SURE
HOW TO CORRECTLY APPLY
YOUR MAKEUP, I SUGGEST
GETTING A MAKEUP
ANALYSIS DONE AT A
COSMETICS BRAND. IT'S
FREE AND A SPECIALIST WILL
MAKE KEY SUGGESTIONS TO
YOU IN TERMS OF APPLYING
MAKEUP IN KEEPING WITH
YOUR FACIAL STRUCTURE
AND COMPLEXION.
TRY SEPHORA, BOBBY
BROWN, MAKE UP FOR EVER,
M·A·C, DIOR, BY TERRY, ETC.

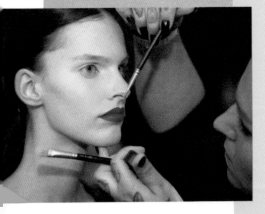

Above: Amanda Murphy – IMG MODELS.

Facing page: Jac Jagaciak – IMG MODELS.

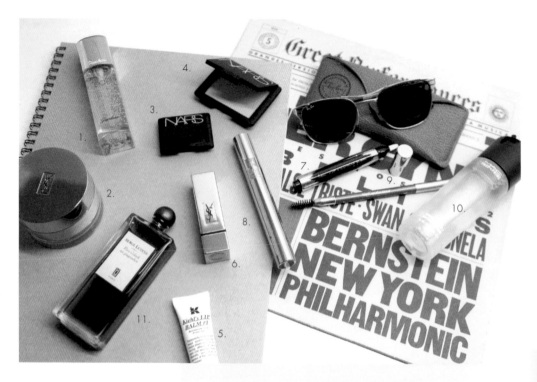

1. Guerlain, l'Or: *makeup base*
2. Yves Saint Laurent, Loose Powder
3. Nars, Eyeshadow
4. Nars, Blush
5. Kiehl's, Lip Balm
6. Yves Saint Laurent, Rouge Pur Couture Satin Radiance Lipstick
7. Yves Saint Laurent, Touche Éclat: (collector's edition)
8. Yves Saint Laurent, Mascara Volume Effet Faux Cils
9. Yves Saint Laurent, Dessin des sourcils
10. MAC, Prep+Prime Fix+
11. Serge Lutens, Five O'Clock au Gingembre
12. Brushes image: Officine Universelle Buly 1803

MAKEUP TOUCH-UP TRICKS
YOU CAN DO THROUGHOUT THE DAY

- Use matte-effect blotting paper to prevent shine.
- Always have a highlighter handy, like Touche Éclat from Yves Saint Laurent.
- Remember to use a pre-base so your makeup lasts longer.
- Moisturize your lips after lunch and put on your lipstick.
- Use a thermal spring water spray to stabilize and refresh makeup.
- Before you go out, comb your eyebrows and add a little mascara and a touch of blush.
- For the evening, to your daytime makeup you can add a darker shadow to the upper eyelid for a smoky look that intensifies your eyes.

MY **10-MINUTE** PERFECT **HAIR** ROUTINE

KEY STEPS
FOR A PERFECT HAIRDO

- Depending on its texture and length, wash your hair three to four times a week.
- Dry your hair with your head upside down. Wrap a towel around it until the water is well absorbed.
- For good volume: with your head upside down, fluff up the roots with good strong brush strokes, then lift your head and set your hairstyle with a spray.
- Lots of products are available to style or smooth the hair. There is hair spray, of course, as well as gel, wax, mousse, and hairgum. Try them and choose what suits you best.
- If your hair is prone to oiliness, use a dry shampoo on the roots at the end of the day (*see* Day 7).

Having a great haircut and beautiful color is key: it structures the face and contributes to the elegance of your look. Make no mistake, the most "natural" hairstyles you see on models are in fact very carefully styled!

Styling your hair well in ten minutes is actually possible, no matter what kind of hair you have.

With my short hair, I usually use no-rinse conditioner after washing it. Since I'm too lazy to blow-dry my hair, I flatten it back with wax so it can take on shape as the morning goes by. I often wear a bow or "flower" barrette in my hair—which my friend Karuna Balloo does a gorgeous job of crafting.

So, having a healthy glow and a good hairstyle is a way of presenting yourself to the world. The idea of "getting gorgeous" is in our genes like the will to live.

Being alive, moving about, being seductive and charming is LIFE itself. So go for it!

09

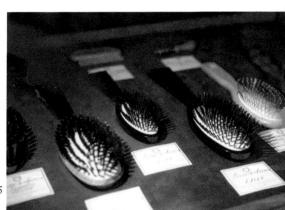

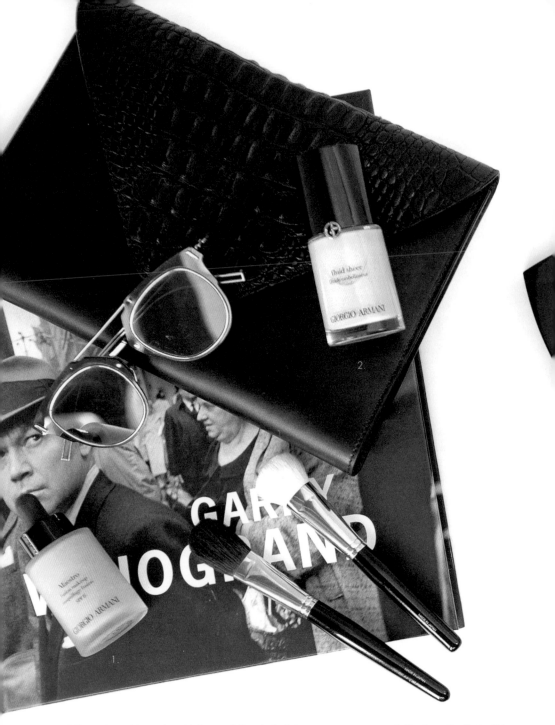

1. Giorgio Armani, Maestro: *fusion blush*

2. Giorgio Armani, Fluid Sheer: *foundation*

3. Chanel, Loose Powder

4. Diptyque, Philosykos: *eau de parfum*

5. Shiseido, Bio-Performance:
   glow revival serum

6. Nars, Radiant Creamy Concealer

7. Giorgio Armani, Eyes to Kill Mascara

8. Dior, Rouge Dior Couture Color

9. Giorgio Armani, Applicator Eyeshaper

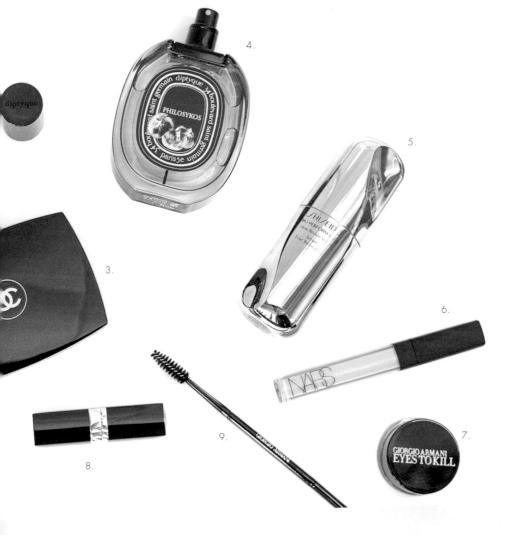

SURVIVAL **KIT**

In my toiletry bag I keep:
- A mirror
- Lip balm or lipstick
- Mascara
- Makeup remover wipes
- Deodorant wipes
- Blush
- Eye shadow

- Moisturizing hand cream
- Hand cleanser gel
- Mini toothbrush with mini toothpaste
- Bobby pins + hair bands
- A mini hairbrush or comb

HOW DO YOU LOOK AFTER MASTERING YOUR NEW BEAUTY ROUTINE? POST A PICTURE!
#getgorgeous, #beautychallenge21

JONATHAN SANCHEZ

MY HAIR & MAKEUP ARTIST

(INSTAGRAM: @JONATHANSANCHEZ_ART)

He's been doing my hair and makeup now for a few years, especially when I attend big events. He also does this for Erin O'Connor, Aymeline Valade, and Lara Stone on a regular basis. So I asked him to give you a few of his professional recommendations:

What's your golden rule for makeup?
I like this quote from Shu Uemura: "Beautiful makeup starts with beautiful skin."

What are your secrets for a flawless complexion?
Makeup base is for covering imperfections but it must always allow the texture of the skin to show. So be careful about over-coverage and a mask effect with foundation.

When you choose your foundation and its shade, always apply it to a clean face. Place a small amount of the product on the jawbone and chin: the zone covered must be the same color as the skin on your neck.

You can find many textures on the market. My favorites are more fluid, like M·A·C's Face and Body foundation, which covers small imperfections but gives a very natural, luminous finish.

Always remember to apply your base to well-moisturized skin and spread the product from the middle of the face toward the outside. You can also use a pre-base. Shu Uemura's Immediate Radiance Skin Perfecting Cream is ideal for making your base more luminous.

I always use a brush, which is more precise than fingers. I swear by M·A·C's 190SH Foundation Brush, which I dampen a little before using with thermal spring water, for guaranteed luminosity.

How do you get perfect red lips?
The most important thing, before putting on any old lipstick, is to have well moisturized, smooth lips. Do a scrub if necessary to remove dry skin.

Apply a bit of your foundation to the lip contours so that your red lipstick makes a perfect line.

Use a lip pencil to define the contour, which will keep your red from running and

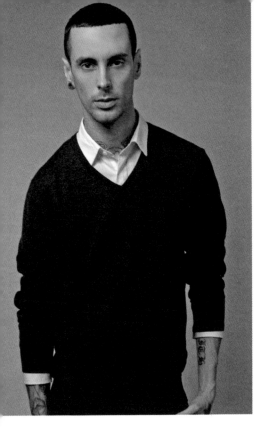

circles—and the upper eyelid, then I smudge it with my fingers from the inside toward the temples.

I apply a nude, matte eye shadow on the upper eyelid and I spread it up a little.

Then I take a nacre eyeshadow like M·A·C's Nylon, and dab a bit of light onto the inner corner of the eye in very small, well-smudged amounts, and also use it very lightly on the outer edge of the eyebrow arch.

Use a lash curler, my favorite is from Laura Mercier.

Apply mascara, being careful to spread it evenly from the base of the lashes toward the tips. Make sure the brush does not contain too much product. The one I like best is Diorshow mascara. Maybelline's Great Lash mascara is also good.

To finish I apply a glow boosting cream such as Diorshow maximizer to the temples, smudging it towards the top of the cheekbones.

What's your golden rule for hair?

There are two:

Like for the skin, what's key to a good hairstyle is to take good care of your hair, using a shampoo and mask suited to your hair type.

It is very important to have a true haircut, otherwise it's difficult to style the hair.

What are you favorite hair products?

To avoid the frizzies I love Redkin's Frizz Dismiss FPF 40 Control Cream.

To protect the fibers before blow-drying I use Redken's Pillow Proof Primer.

To give hair texture and fullness, I like Kevin.Murphy's Night.Rider matte texture paste.

To keep colored hair from splitting, I recommend Redken's Anti-Snap in its Extrême line.

To model and sculpt your hair with a matte effect: Sebastian's Molding Mud.

To moisturize, protect, and make your hair shinier and easy to style you can use Sebastian's Potion 9.

creasing into the nearby fine lines. My favorite is the Nars Cosmetics Lip Liner Pencil Jungle Red. Ever equipped with your pencil, smudge the contour line toward the inside of the lips.

Finally, apply your lipstick, preferably with a thin brush, for a more precise effect. My favorite is M·A·C's Ruby Woo, one of the matte reds that holds longest.

If you want a glossier effect, wear a gloss like Nars Cosmetics Lip Gloss Scandal over your lipstick.

How do you like to do eye makeup?

I like simplicity for eye makeup. It's important for them to look bright and natural. Brush your eyebrows so the shape is good. You can even apply a clear gel. I use Dior's Brow Styler Gel.

Use a highlighter, like the Yves Saint Laurent Touche Éclat. I dab small touches of it on the lower eye area—the under-eye

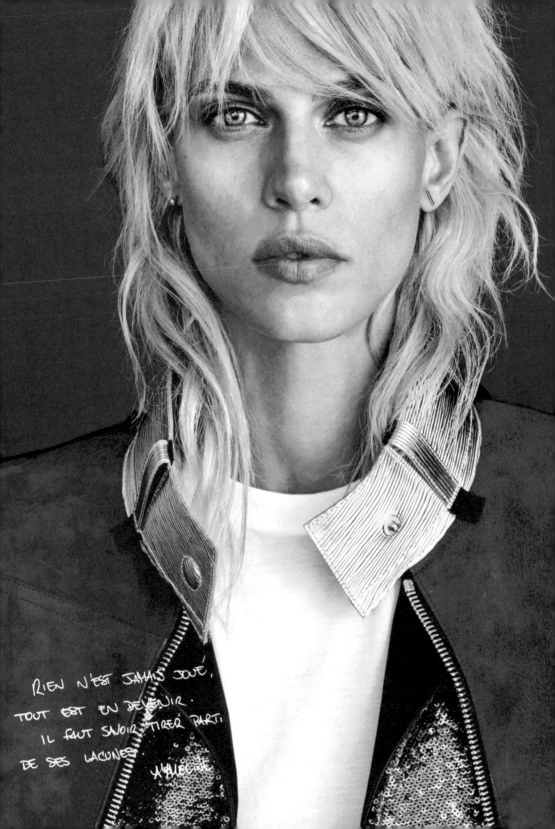

RIEN N'EST JAMAIS JOUÉ,
TOUT EST EN DEVENIR.
IL FAUT SAVOIR TIRER PARTI
DE SES LACUNES.

Aymeline Valade

AGE: 31
PROFESSION: Model
FIRST JOB: The Balenciaga fashion show by Nicolas Ghesquière
YOUR FAVORITE PHOTO OF YOURSELF: It was never published, but it was by Mert & Marcus for the Giorgio Armani campaign
ASTROLOGICAL SIGN: Libra
DISTINGUISHING FEATURE: Piercing blue eyes
WHAT CAN'T YOU LIVE WITHOUT: A good night's sleep
WHAT DO YOU DO AS A SPECIAL TREAT FOR YOURSELF: Spend good times with my friends
YOUR THREE SIGNATURE WARDROBE PIECES: Black jeans, a beautiful pair of shoes with personality, fine jewelry
THREE MUST-HAVE BEAUTY PRODUCTS: The Soy Face Cleanser from Fresh cosmetics, an organic, musky rose plant oil, and a healthy organic diet
YOUR PERFUME: The smell of my skin; I don't wear perfume
WHO IS YOUR IDOL: Josephine Baker, a woman who swam against the tide and liberated herself
WHAT BOOK IS ON YOUR NIGHTSTAND: *The Finger and the Moon* by Alejandro Jodorowsky
YOUR LUCKY CHARM: I don't have any. I don't think objects in themselves bring luck, but that people do.
LESS OR MORE: Less!
YOUR MOTTO: "Work it."
YOUR ADVICE FOR READERS (facing page): Nothing is ever set in stone, everything possible. You have to know how to make the most of your weaknesses.

Is it a challenge for you to do your makeup and style your hair in 10 minutes? No, it's quick when you know yourself well.
What's the best makeup advice you've ever received? To use highlighter (a makeup method that enables you to bring out the facial structure with light and shadow).
The key makeup items you carry in your handbag? Mascara, lash curler, highlighter, blush, and a concealer just to cover a few imperfections.
Are you always made up? No, only for events. If you wear makeup every day, you have no room to maneuver to create a "wow" effect the day you need to.
A recent beauty makeover that you liked? My latest cover for *Air France Madame*.
For or against sophistication? For! Sophistication has nothing to do with the luxuriousness of clothes or with the idea of "too much." It's the attention you pay to details.

DAY

10

GETTING

Dressed

IN 10 MINUTES

SAVE TIME

SHOW ME WHAT **YOU'RE WEARING**, I'LL TELL YOU WHO YOU ARE!

"Wearing clothes and shoes that fit: now that's wisdom."

Horace

Who hasn't had a day ruined due to inappropriate clothes that weren't carefully thought out? Spending the day badly dressed because you pulled the wrong thing out of your closet is unbearable. I have been in situations where I didn't pay attention to my look, only to find myself meeting important people: a nightmare! Thinking about your style and clothes in advance is to rid yourself of worry. Preparing your clothes the night before or early in the week might seem like a useless discipline, but in fact, it's a real timesaver. Clothing is like armor. Feeling good and beautiful is a time-saver: once that is sorted out, you can think about other things.

Being well dressed is not a superficial act and I don't believe in the saying, "The clothes don't make the man." Clothes define us socially, provide information about who we are and the emotional state in which we find ourselves. Wearing flashy clothes or a go-anywhere uniform does not produce the same effect on the people around you. Although there are more important things than clothing, I am nevertheless convinced that the way we appear to others is critical. In modeling agencies, we spend our time explaining to young women that we are their first customers. We are the ones they must convince to promote them, well before the casting directors they will meet in their career. As the boss, I always asked them to introduce themselves to the team as they would to a casting director: all dressed up and in high heels! You should do the same!

Now that we have selected your basics (*see* Day 4) and sorted through your clothes (*see* Day 5), we can come up with different looks for every day of the week and special events.

IT'S ALL A **QUESTION** OF BEING **ORGANIZED**

It's very simple, really. You just have to prepare things ahead of time, not at the last minute. Pick out the key events of your week, and, depending on the season, decide on your different looks.

On a daily basis: You're in a hurry and have no time to waste choosing your clothes. The best advice to keep from tearing your hair out every morning is to choose a uniform! Yes, you heard me, a uniform. Obviously I don't mean for you to turn yourself into a GI Jane or a cop. Your uniform is in fact your go-to look, the one that seems best adapted to your work and the one that makes you feel "confident." It could be a navy blazer, jeans, a loose-fitting cream-colored blouse, and pair of heels you feel comfortable wearing, for example. So instead of changing your look every day, with the accompanying loss of time and style risks involved, opt for repetition: an outfit that you know ahead of time works very well and that you can vary slightly, from one day to the next.

Important days: when I want to mark an occasion, make a splash at a party or dinner, or simply knock out my boyfriend. Without question, this requires preparation; it must be thought out at least one day ahead of time. Try on your outfit to make sure you feel at ease in it and that everything is impeccably clean and ironed. It is also the moment to choose your accessories (*see* Day 13). The time you'll have spent, the day before an important event, on creating a ready-to-go look that is well organized in your closet creates free time that you can spend getting gorgeous on the day in question. There is nothing worse than wearing a gorgeous dress and not having enough time to do your hair and makeup.

At my house, the preparation sessions take place on Sunday. I come up with about ten looks ahead of time.

DEFINE YOUR UNIFORM

Apart from the convenience, by creating your uniform, you'll help bolster your image and style, like Karl Lagerfeld who for several years has worn variations of the same look.

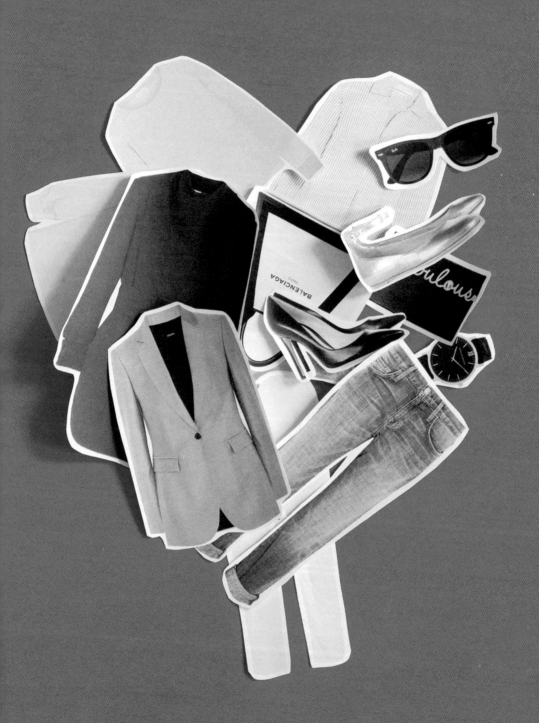

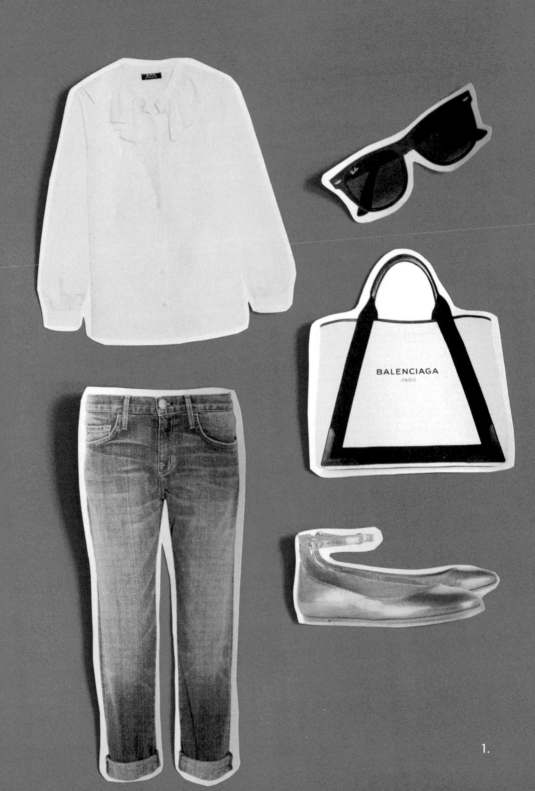

1.

A FEW **READY-TO-WEAR LOOKS**

1 FOR A **CASUAL** (OR RELAXED) LOOK, CHOOSE:

• A white shirt/T-shirt beneath a sweater
• Beige/khaki pants or jeans
• Flat shoes: derbies or ballet flats
or
• A chic blouse
• Slim jeans
• A gorgeous pair of sneakers

2 FOR A SUBTLE AND TASTEFULLY **CHIC** LOOK, YOU CAN WEAR:

• A black men's jacket
• A silk top or tank top
• Jeans
• Stilettos
or
• A black jumpsuit
• Accessorized with a fabulous brooch or elegant bracelet
• Platform shoes

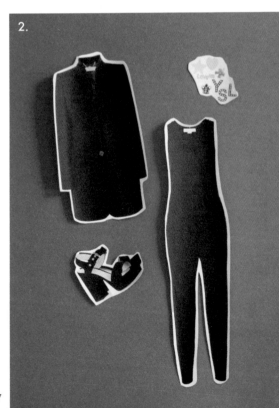

2.

117

TO **HELP YOU** WITH THIS EXERCISE

- Start by thinking of an item from your closet. Once you've made your choice, try combining it with other clothes.
- Don't hesitate to layer clothes and mix different lengths.

- To save time you can also take photos of your looks! Get inspiration from shopping websites featuring ready-to-wear looks.

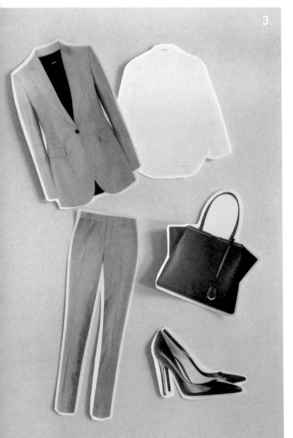

3.

3 FOR A **BUSINESS** LOOK, OPT FOR DARK COLORS (BLACK, NAVY, OR GRAY):

- A suit or skirt
- A belt (gold, for example) to highlight your waist
- 1½- to 3-inch (4-7 cm) heels, ideal for work

or
- A loose blouse
- Men's black pants with cuffs rolled up
- Heels or ballet flats

4 FOR A **DINNER-IN-THE-CITY** LOOK:

- The famous little black dress, worn over bare legs
- Sandals with heels

or
- A clingy top with a pencil skirt
- Heels

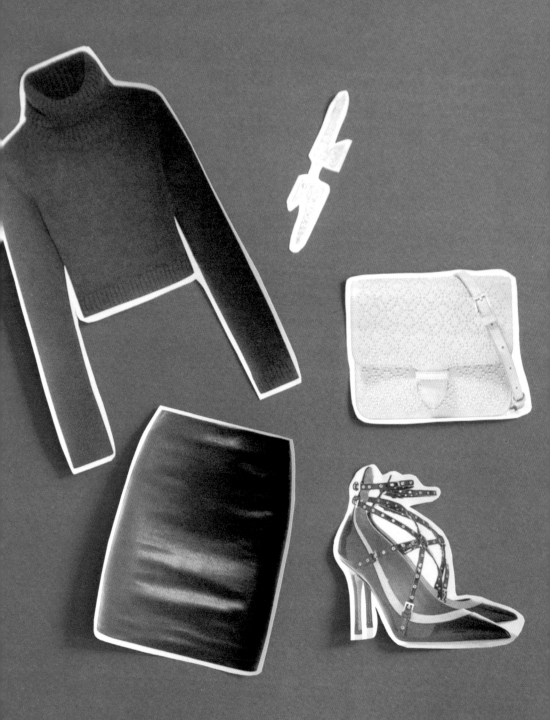

4.

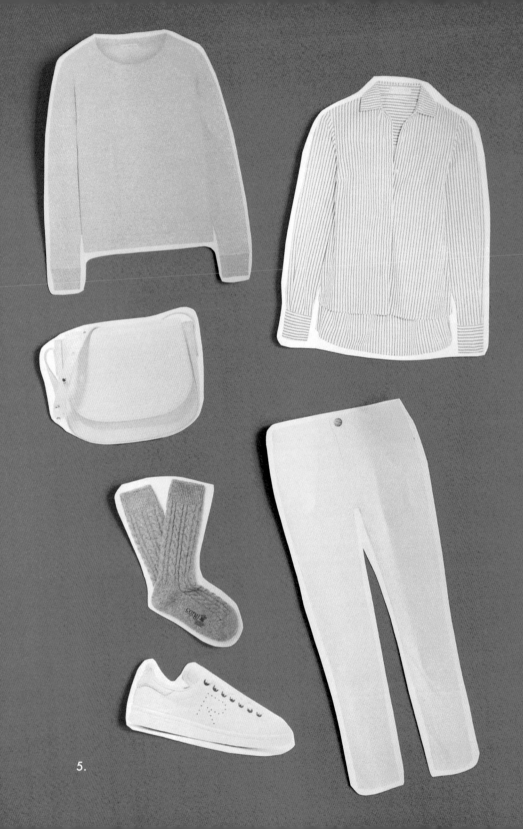

5.

5
FOR A **CASUAL FRIDAY** LOOK THAT'S COOL BUT CHIC:

• Gray or navy sweatshirt
• Jeans
• A pair of Stan Smith™ sneakers
or
• A denim shirt
• Jeans with a big, brown leather belt
• Ballerina flats

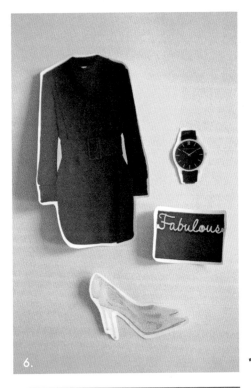

6.

6
FOR A **ROMANTIC DATE**, BE SEXY:

• A dress fitted at the waist or a short skirt (colorful or patterned)
• A small hand-held clutch
• Stilettos
or
• A blouse tucked into slim jeans
• High heels, again!

7
FOR A SPECIAL **SOIRÉE**, DARE TO WEAR BRIGHT COLORS AND DIFFERENT CUTS:

• A bustier top with shorts
• High but comfortable heels (so your feet won't hurt if you dance!)
or
• A form-fitting T-shirt with a miniskirt
• Boots or platform shoes

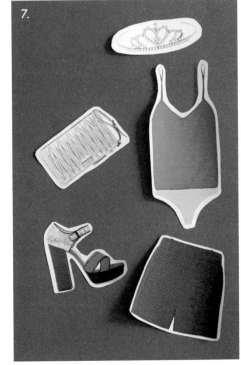

7.

POST YOUR FAVORITE OUTFIT.
#getgorgeous, #beautychallenge21

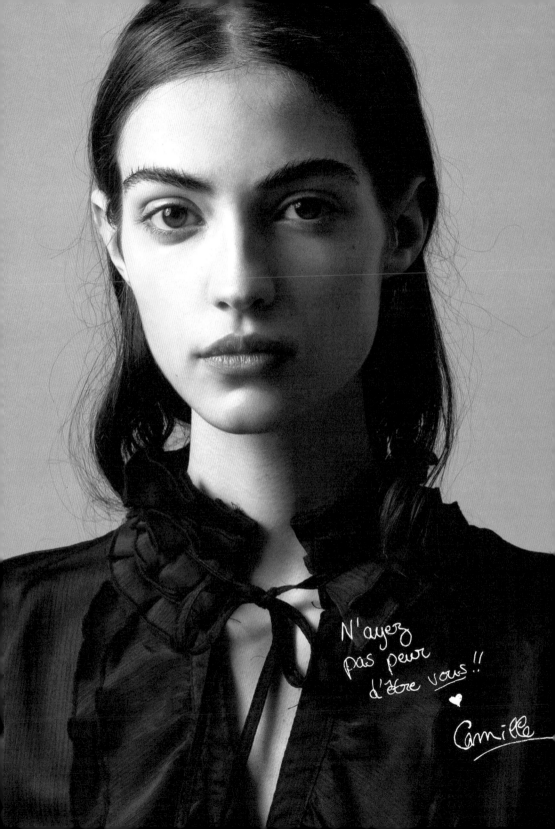

N'ayez
pas peur
d'être vous !!
♥
Camille

Camille Huret

AGE: 18
PROFESSION: Model
FIRST JOB: Valentino lookbook in Rome
YOUR FAVORITE PHOTO OF YOURSELF: My first *Crash* cover, my first show, photos with friends and family
ASTROLOGICAL SIGN: Aquarius
DISTINGUISHING FEATURE: My eyes and eyebrows, my usual good mood
WHAT CAN'T YOU LIVE WITHOUT: My family and friends who are my support. And, being on the go, cooking and my Adidas—for running when I'm late.
WHAT DO YOU DO AS A SPECIAL TREAT FOR YOURSELF: I cook, take care of myself, and see friends
YOUR THREE SIGNATURE WARDROBE PIECES: Sandro bomber jacket, leather pants, shirt sewn by my grandmother
THREE MUST-HAVE BEAUTY PRODUCTS: Bioderma cleansing lotion before bed, magic Eucerin *Aquaphor* cold cream—you can use it for everything (especially blisters), M·A·C lipstick
YOUR PERFUME: I don't have a regular one, but I love Chanel's Cuir de Russie
WHO IS YOUR IDOL: People who fight for and teach others to fight for their dreams
WHAT BOOK IS ON YOUR NIGHTSTAND: I put my detective stories aside for Lena Dunham's funny and touching *Not That Kind of Girl*
YOUR LUCKY CHARM: Nothing specific; when I feel good in my clothes and my head, I'm ready for anything
LESS OR MORE: You can never have enough rings!
YOUR MOTTO: "Don't stop until you're proud" or "Never underestimate your ability to fulfill your dreams." Jérôme Jarre's advice for believing in yourself and staying positive.
YOUR ADVICE FOR READERS: Confidence comes with time. Be yourself, with no window dressing, and you'll respect yourself and be respected by others. Get to it!

Do you panic in front of your closet every morning? It depends on the day, but generally I have figured out a day ahead of time what I'm going to wear, so I can get up as late as possible. If I panic, it's because I've changed clothes at the last minute because I don't like them anymore, and then it's a race to find the right thing....

Do you have a "uniform look"? I regularly change my style. I like to diversify my looks and when I don't know what to wear, I put on my Schott leather jacket, my imitation leather jeans, and my ankle boots or Adidas when I want to feel more comfortable.

Do you borrow clothes from the man in your life? From my dad! His sweaters, or very often, his scarves, which by now are no longer really his!

What do you do when you have no time to change clothes before you go out in the evening? I always find the time to change clothes. Otherwise, I would bet on matte lipstick or mascara, with a natural look for the rest. Then go!

Do you dress for yourself or for others? Generally I dress for myself. I like to dress in keeping with my mood, no matter what other people think. Your way of dressing reflects a part of your personality. You don't have to be super dressed up to be a good person!

Facing page: Don't be afraid to be you!

01
02
03
04
05
06
07
08
09
10
11
12
13
14
15
16
17
18
19
20
21

11

DESIGNING MY SIGNATURE

Scent

MY OWN UNIQUE FRAGRANCE

THE **PERFUME** THAT REFLECTS MY **PERSONALITY**

"He who ruled scent
ruled the hearts of men."

Patrick Süskind, *Perfume: The Story of a Murderer*

Who has ever done a better job of describing the pleasant feeling of associating a memory with a savor or scent than Marcel Proust, writing about the madeleine in *Swann's Way*? For Proust's narrator, dipping a madeleine in tea evoked childhood memories of another madeleine dipped in tea at his Aunt Léonie's.

Now that I'm in my forties and have some life experience under my belt, my mind is filled with many "Proustian madeleines": the unique smell of the Saponifère soap shop on Rue Bonaparte, where I used to spend time after school; the scent of the perfume Égoïste that my first love wore; the smell of freshly cut grass that always reminds me of my grandfather mowing the lawn. Then there's Clinique's Élixir, which takes me back to a memory of my mother when I was ten. And it took me ages to find my father's cologne, which reminds me of his morning ritual splashing it on head-to-toe in the bathroom.

I've always liked wearing perfume as a result.

The first perfume I ever received as a gift was Ô de Lancôme. I made a special collage about it.

Since then I have never stopped changing perfumes. Each reflects a different moment of my life. When I was pregnant with my second son Tao, I wore L'Artisan Parfumeur's Bois Farine, and now it is the reminder of that unique time in my life.

For the past few years I've enjoyed mixing and matching fragrances, and I love trying new ones.

We all love perfume, and even people who never wear it don't realize they are actually sporting one of the greatest of all: the scent of their own skin, the very same that Jean-Baptiste Grenouille, the hero of Patrick Süskind's novel *Perfume*, spent his life trying to capture.

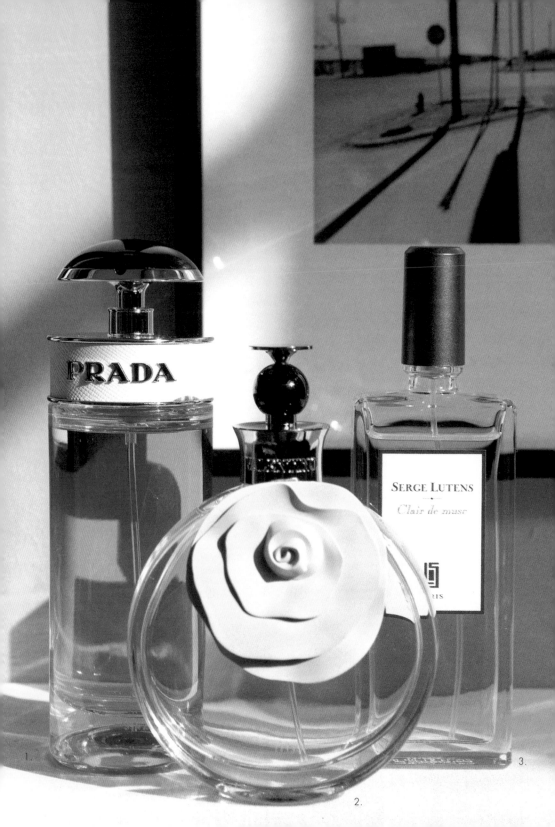

1.

PRADA

2.

3.

SERGE LUTENS
•
Clair de musc

THE SCENT
OF A WOMAN

That said, it's true that wearing perfume is not entirely straightforward. Some people are great at it, leaving such a characteristic scent lingering in the air as they go by that we call it their OLFACTORY SIGNATURE, or *sillage* in French. Haven't you ever perceived someone's presence from their perfume? The ability to leave the air filled with one's scent is very primal, but it's also the height of elegance, a sign of true power, and a real weapon of seduction. In a way, your fragrance is the extension of your aura. A means of making your presence extend beyond your body, of making it felt in a wider area, a very subtle way of entering into communication with others.

Today's objective is to give you the key to finding YOUR OWN olfactory signature and to teach you to use it as a formidable weapon.

So you'll have to immerse yourself for a while in the vast world of perfume and understand a few rules to help guide you along.

Facing page:
1. Prada, Candy l'Eau: *eau de toilette*
2. Valentino, Valentina: *eau de parfum*
3. Serge Lutens, Clair de Musc

A REAL SCIENCE

We can't create a scented olfactory signature without broaching the subject of perfume composition and concentration. Perfume, as you probably know, is made up of essential oils diluted with alcohol. But did you know that perfume formulas are different depending on whether the fragrance is a perfume extract or a light eau de parfum?

To understand perfume, you have to remember what is called the "fragrance pyramid," which is structured as follows:
- Top notes: the most volatile notes, the ones you smell right when you put on a perfume and that fade after a few minutes.
- The heart notes: these last several hours and are the main ones that characterize the perfume.
- The base notes: these build up slowly and can last several days.

THERE ARE THREE
MAJOR PRODUCT TYPES

- Extrait de parfum (also called "parfum" or "extrait"): rich in base notes, it lasts several hours. It's essential for a pronounced fragrance signature. Careful, though—it can stain your clothes.

The more top notes a fragrance has, the fresher and more evanescent it will be, and the more quickly it will wear off. The more base notes it has, the richer and more sensual the fragrance will be.

1. Guerlain, Aqua Allegoria Pamplelune: eau de toilette
2. Nina Ricci, L'Air du Temps: eau de parfum
3. Guerlain, L'Heure Bleue: eau de parfum

- Eau de parfum: similar to extrait, it contains lots of heart and base notes, but it wears off more quickly.
- Eau de toilette: rich in very volatile top notes, its presence is more pronounced for you than for other people. It fades very quickly.

To complete our review of the technical aspects of perfume, here is a short list of the major fragrance families:

1. **Citrus:** bergamot, lemon, orange, mandarin, grapefruit, orange blossom, and neroli. These are dynamic and energizing notes.
2. **Amber:** rose, jasmine, violet, amber, sandalwood, and vanilla. Captivating and mysterious.
3. **Aromatic:** sage, rosemary, thyme, and lavender, to which are added citrus and spicy notes. These create strong, fresh fragrances.
4. **Floral:** rose, jasmine, ylang-ylang, tuberose, and carnation. Particularly feminine.
5. **Leather:** tobacco, smoke, fur, wood. This family has the least number of perfumes. The notes are more masculine, but they can give women character.
6. **Chypré:** oak moss, bergamot, jasmine, rose, patchouli, labdanum, and animal notes. Very persistent, with a strong character.
7. **Fougère:** lavender, oak moss, woody notes, coumarine, and bergamot. These are the vetiver fragrances, which are extremely masculine.

It's really all about taste and knowledge of the subject, and it's very subjective and sentimental. There's no such thing as good and bad taste here, just very personal choices.

Whether you like floral, coppery scents or simply aromatic notes matters little. What's key is how you wear your perfume; that's what makes all the difference.

Like for your skin and hair, we suggest you create YOUR OWN ROUTINE, a succession of steps and small indulgences that will make your fragrance signature UNIQUE.

Coco Chanel, again, once artfully said:

"You should wear perfume wherever you want to be kissed."

Often we limit ourselves to spraying perfume onto our neck or wrists. The secret to a successful fragrance signature lies in wearing just a little bit of perfume but in plenty of different places.

Emphasize the "hot spots" in particular, your pulse points: the base (front) and the nape (back) of the neck, the wrists, behind the ear, between the breasts, the ankles, the lower back, and the navel. Throughout the day, your pulsating skin and the warmth emanating from these spots will diffuse the fragrance you've dabbed on.

When you're in a very big hurry, Estée Lauder has a very useful tip: "Spray a cloud of perfume in front of you and then walk into it."

Your body is not the only place you can wear perfume. *Sillage,* as we've already mentioned, refers to a trail of fragrance that lingers as you go by. Perfuming your clothes is an important step in creating your *sillage.*

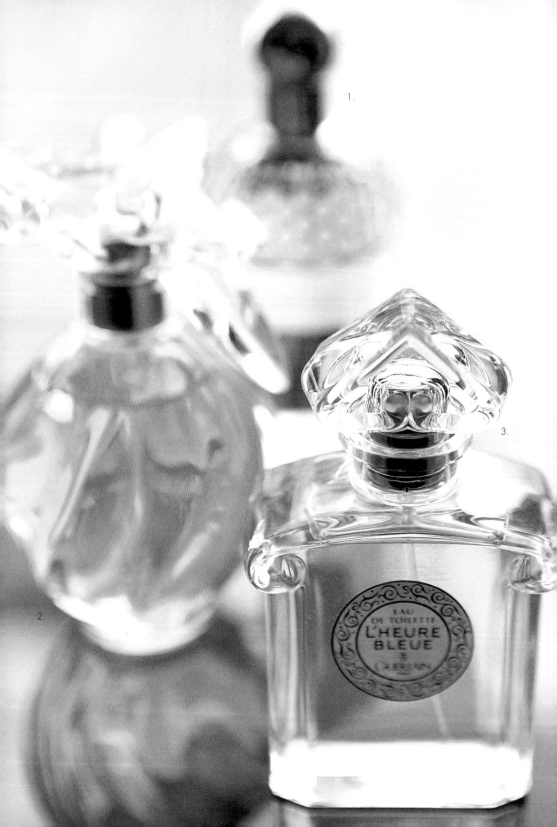

1.

2.

3.

EAU DE TOILETTE
L'HEURE
BLEUE
GUERLAIN

1. Narciso Rodriguez, Narciso: *eau de parfum*
2. Chloé, Chloé: *eau de toilette*
3. Narciso Rodriguez, For Her: *eau de parfum*
4. Giorgio Armani, Sì: *eau de toilette*
5. Dior, J'adore Eau Lumière: *eau de toilette*

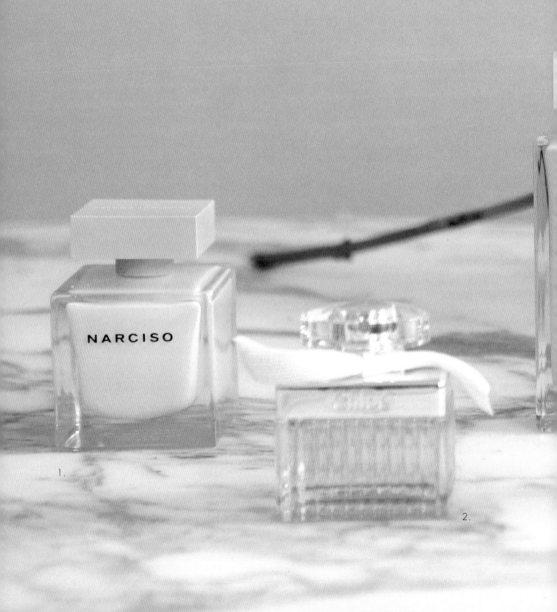

1.

2.

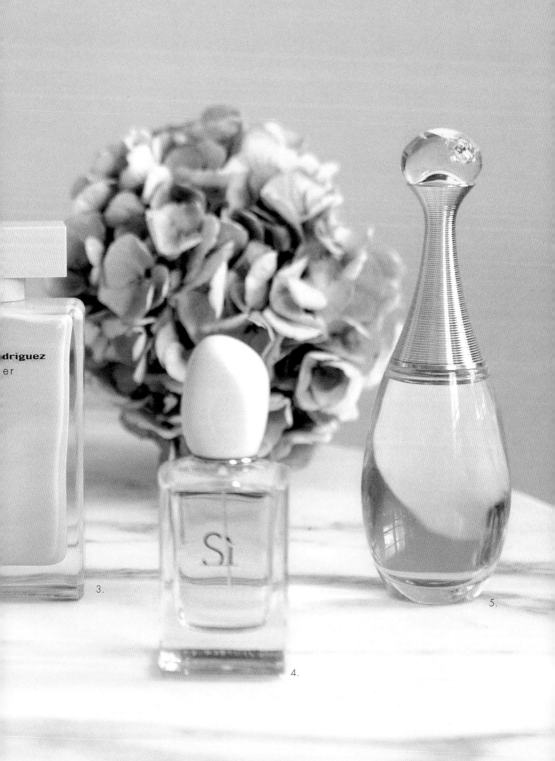

driguez
er

3.

Si

4.

5.

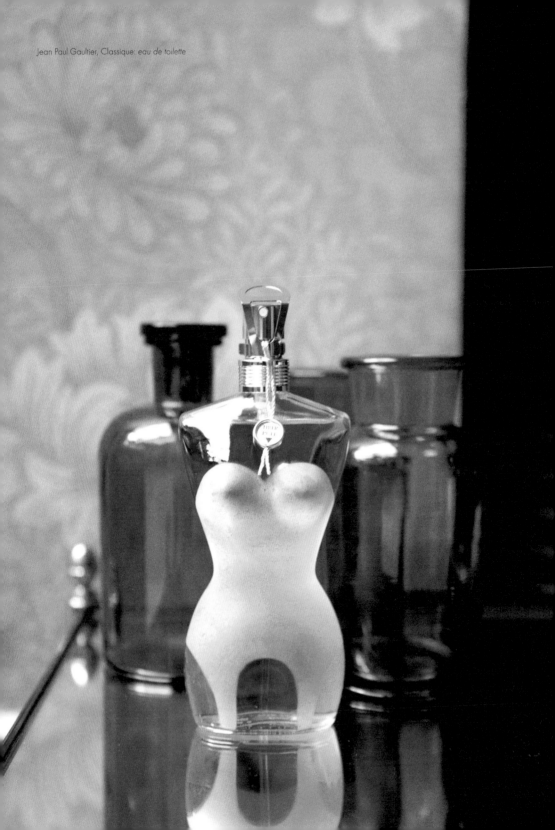
Jean Paul Gaultier, Classique: eau de toilette

ARE YOU A
ONE-PERFUME
WOMAN?

It's time for a word about perfume loyalty. We're all tempted to change perfumes often, and the vast selection available offers even more of an invitation to do so. Yet be aware that creating a fragrance signature is also a matter of repetition. No one memorizes the perfume of someone who changes fragrances too often. And if you perfume your clothes, either accidentally or on purpose, don't forget that the famous base notes last several days and they could create an unpleasant combination when you switch from one fragrance to another.

I can't do enough to recommend loyalty. It's a bit like a love story. So don't hesitate to perfume some of your clothes, notably the most portable, like foulards and scarves, and also coat linings and pants cuffs. If you want to be over-the-top elegant, you can sprinkle a few drops of perfume into your lingerie wash cycle, soak a hanky to carry in your pocket, or rub a few drops into your handbag.

Finally, remember you can also spritz your closet or armoire with perfume (*see* Day 5) or you can mist a little fragrance on a radiator to scent a room.

Let's close this chapter by talking about perfume spin-offs, which also help create a real fragrance signature. We're talking about the ancillary products in perfume lines, such as body milk, soap, shower gel, shampoo, and scented oil. These will subtly enhance the presence of your fragrance. But going back to our mantra "less is more": it's not about overdoing it with perfume or spraying it on too often, but of managing plenty of tiny details that will make you unique. All the little scented notes you'll have spread here and there become silently seductive calling cards.

11

For a **lasting fragrance signature**, I spray a bit of perfume:
- On the base of my neck
- On the nape of my neck
- Behind my ear
- Between my breasts
- On my wrists
- On my lower back
- On my navel
- On my ankles
- On my clothes

WHICH PERFUME DID YOU CHOOSE TODAY?
#getgorgeous, #beautychallenge21

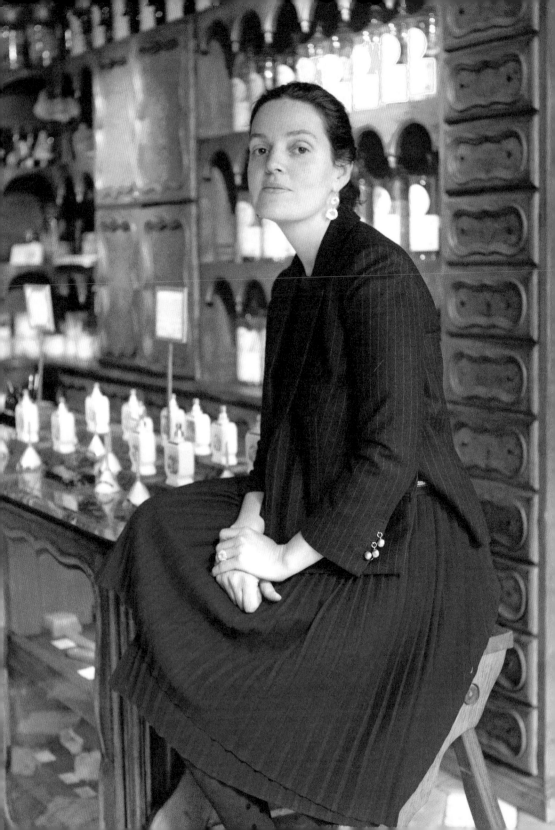

Victoire de Taillac

AGE: 41
PROFESSION: Founder of Officine Universelle Buly 1803
FIRST JOB: Publicist at Colette
YOUR FAVORITE PHOTO OF YOURSELF: With my children
ASTROLOGICAL SIGN: Capricorn
DISTINGUISHING FEATURE: Lots of hair
WHAT CAN'T YOU LIVE WITHOUT: Flowers
WHAT DO YOU DO AS A SPECIAL TREAT FOR YOURSELF: Spend the day outside gardening
YOUR THREE SIGNATURE WARDROBE PIECES: Jacket, dress, Azzedine Alaïa oxfords
THREE MUST-HAVE BEAUTY PRODUCTS: Floral water, cream, and oil
YOUR PERFUME: Eau Triple Miel d'Angleterre, by Buly 1803
WHO IS YOUR IDOL: Virginia Woolf
WHAT BOOK IS ON YOUR NIGHTSTAND: Alexandre Dumas' *Dictionary of Cuisine*
YOUR LUCKY CHARM: A Japanese gris-gris
LESS OR MORE: Less
YOUR MOTTO: "One for all, all for one."
YOUR ADVICE FOR READERS (right): Highlight what you love about yourself, don't try to hide what you hate. Perfect as you are!

What is your Proustian madeleine (a fragrant childhood memory)? The smell of red currant jelly while my great aunt was cooking it.
What was your first perfume? Nina Ricci's L'Air du Temps.
Is it important to have a signature fragrance? No, it's fun to play with scents, to combine them and change them.
Is it important to favor perfumes with natural essences? No, you should place emphasis on what is appealing to you and choose good perfume houses.
What perfume ad made an impact on you? All the Serge Lutens campaigns.
Do you have to be loyal to your perfume? No.
Apart from your body, what should you perfume? Your closets.
What perfume would you borrow from men? The colognes.

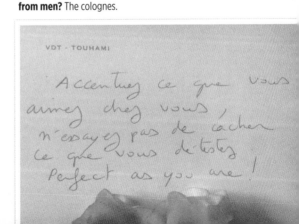

VDT · TOUHAMI

Accentuez ce que vous aimez chez vous, n'essayez pas de cacher ce que vous détestez. Perfect as you are!

12

CHOOSING MY

Shoes

FLATS VS. HEELS, IT DEPENDS ON THE OCCASION

WE'RE ALL **CRAZY** ABOUT **SHOES**

"Wearing your dreams on your feet is one way to start making your dreams come true."

Roger Vivier

Careful now. We are about to enter into one of the most irrational zones: SHOES.

We all have an ambiguous relationship with shoes. Above all as an accessory, they keep our feet on the ground, no pun intended. Thanks to them we can move around and conquer the world. But they also drive us crazy. Many of us can spend wild sums of money on them, accumulating and collecting them with the sole aim of owning them. There is no logic to it, no clear reasoning when it comes to shoes.

When shoes are too new, too small, or have heels that are too high, we often associate them with pain. Also with pleasure and seductiveness, due to their erotic, even fetish potential. After all there's a reason

Christian Louboutin's red soles are such a hit. The red alone is the very symbol of pain and pleasure, two opposing ideas that go hand in hand. Shoes also serve a real social function. As Manolo Blahnik says, with a dash of humor: "Men tell me that I've saved their marriages. It costs them a fortune in shoes, but it's cheaper than a divorce. So I'm still useful, you see."

Choosing shoes can be tricky, triggering passionate discussion and a clash of opinions. Whether you're a heels addict like I am or you swear by flats, the key thing is to find the shoe that fits!

Cutting to the chase, whatever your taste, here are a few rules that will help you choose the right pair of shoes.

I'M CRAZY ABOUT
HEELS. HIGH HEELS.
(I'M TALKING
ABOUT MYSELF, HERE!)

Heels represent the ultimate women's accessory, the one modern men have never been able to expropriate, in spite of Jean Paul Gaultier's attempts.

I admire women who spend their entire life in high heels and would never dream of wearing anything else. However, though I am in love with heels, I'm not an extremist. I refuse to submit to the torture of an overly uncomfortable pair; it's just not necessary.

Yet I must admit that when I have an important business meeting or simply want to seduce someone, heels are a must. No matter their height. Even a small inch can change everything. It's psychological, mostly. A bit like wearing a blazer that will give you a certain look. Heels give you a different demeanor, gait, curve, and way of carrying your head. There's no point in lying. Wearing heels often requires effort, but it makes you reach beyond your limits. It's a way of stimulating you, of putting yourself a little at risk, of challenging your femininity.

More simply, heels are the most effective way to add height and streamline your legs.

But be careful. Wearing heels is not enough to make you look alluring. On the contrary! I often run into high-heeled women in the street whose gait is really hesitant, even awkward.

Would you be surprised if I told you that one of the first things a beginner model is taught is how to walk? On a catwalk, of course.

That meow-ish slink that is characteristic of the catwalk is rarely innate. Beginner models practice for hours. We even recommend that they watch fashion show videos on YouTube.

Having a beautiful gait in heels is something you can acquire.

If you are ill at ease, the secret is to practice at home, starting over until you can do it correctly. It's worth the trouble.

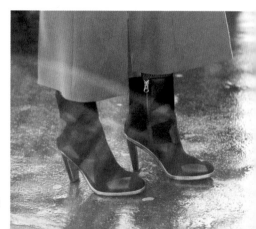

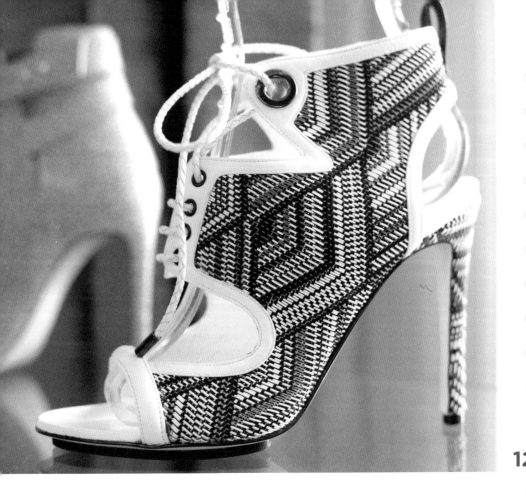

A FEW **RULES** TO FOLLOW

- Never wear shoes with heels either too low or too high.
- Take the time to try on shoes when you buy them, notably to make sure the arch is comfortable. Avoid buying shoes online.
- Favor reasonable heights, from 2–3 inches (5–7 cm) when you are just getting started.
- Have a shoe repairman add a slip-proof pad to the soles of your shoes, which will keep you steadier than a leather insole and will guarantee an easier gait. Slip-proof pads can be purchased at most drugstores and applied at home, too.
- Take your time! You can't run in heels like you do in sneakers.
- Shift your weight to the tips of your toes for balance, and not to the heels, which could create unsteadiness.

HOW TO **CHOOSE** YOUR **HEELS**

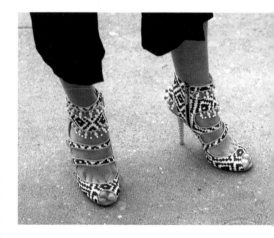

Shoes, and particularly heels, are one feature of a look that always attracts attention. They're a little like your calling card, so there is no room for mediocrity here. In fact it was a queen, and not the least of them, who first brought heels to the kingdom of France. In 1533, Catherine de Médicis had a pair of heeled slippers imported from Florence for her marriage to the duke of Orléans, who was later to become Henry II of France. A symbol of opulence, an object representing sixteenth-century luxury and privilege, heeled slippers lost their stature after the French Revolution and only regained popularity again in the nineteenth century. In the twentieth century, heels took turns looking demure or outlandish, changing to suit women's needs and priorities. Over the centuries, a variety of connotations have been ascribed to heels that were never innocent or devoid of social meaning. So when you decide to wear them, you can't do so halfway.

Here are my rules for choosing the right pair:

1 WHAT **HEIGHT** SHOULD YOUR **HEELS** BE?

For me heels should make a statement, so they are necessarily a bit extreme.

Remember, in fashion we like clear choices that are visually powerful. The bravest of you will want to go for heels higher than 4 inches (10 cm)—preferably without platforms, for a more graceful look—but very low 1 inch (3 cm) heels can also be very sexy. Intermediary heights, around 2 inches (5 cm), are not so great, because the message is not very clear: "I want to wear high heels but I don't really know how."

2 ROUND OR **POINTY TOES**?

This is a question of style. And in fashion, styles change very quickly. Right now I would be ready to spend a fortune to own a pair of the latest very pointy-toed Saint Laurent catwalk stilettos. But what will I think of them in six months? I don't actually know. The only thing I can tell you is that the pointed shapes lend themselves to more of a rock look and rounded toes are more romantic.

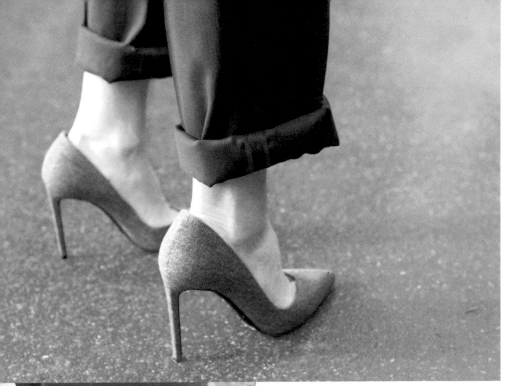

4 CAREFUL ABOUT LOW-CUT FRONTS

(We're not talking neckline here, but toe cleavage) and the curve of your foot. Again, you must try on shoes before buying them. A fabulous-looking pair might not flatter the curve of your foot or it may reveal too much toe. On the other hand, a pair that seems less attractive to you could show off your foot to its best advantage.

3 STILETTOS OR CHUNKY HEELS?

Again, the shape doesn't matter, provided the shoes are worn with confidence. Stiletto heels must be very thin, square heels really solid, and wedges must be real wedges. No matter its shape, a heel must have a clean, streamlined look, with no fancy touches or overly rounded shapes.

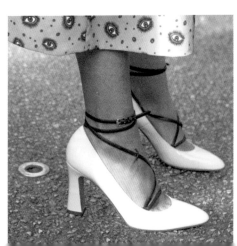

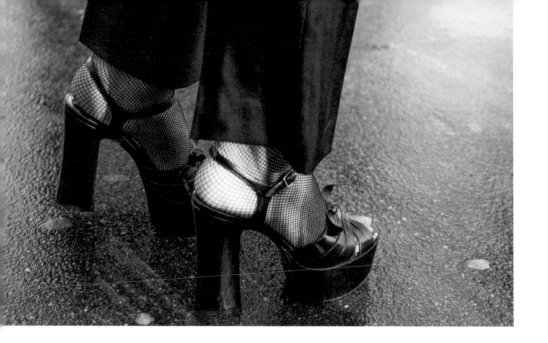

5 INVEST

Heels cannot be mediocre. It's cool to have a pair of inexpensive sneakers like **Vans®** or **Stan Smith**™. But a pair of inexpensive heels remains forever a pair of inexpensive heels. The moral of the story is, if you don't have the means to invest in several pairs, it's better to invest in one very beautiful pair that you wear only occasionally (alternating with flats) and that will be sensational. Fortunately today between sales, discount websites, and vintage shops, you can give in to your dream pair, the pair that will turn you into a real princess.

6 DREAM

Having a good pair of black pumps is a given, but just one pair of heels is not enough. For all the others, please have fun! Buy color, play around with different materials, widen your scope! Heels are one of the best ways to give your look a twist, so don't deprive yourself (*see* Day 16). Front-row stylists at fashion shows get it, outdoing one another with daring, sometimes questionable, but always memorable choices. They go for color, favor materials with a luxurious look like python or alligator (real or fake), and they're not afraid of patent or metallic leather. They foray into metal or precious-wood heels. In short, they rock out.

> Stop thinking the ideal pair is the one that goes with everything. *Au contraire.* The ideal pair is the one you flip over. You see nothing but it. It's so sexy it can liven up a basic look (jean + white T-shirt) all by itself.

I **SWEAR** BY **FLATS**...
(EVEN I WEAR THEM, OCCASIONALLY)

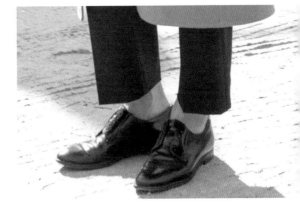

The perfect flats are indisputably men's shoes. Knowing this will help you make the right choice.

Want to look feminine? Go for the heels. Otherwise try models men could wear. You can't go wrong with the following classics:

SNEAKERS
I have developed a major aversion to very complicated, falsely girly, or overly precious sneakers. A pair of sneakers should be simple, almost minimalist, preferably in a basic color and a clear design (not too elegant), which leads us to Nike Air, Adidas Stan Smith™, and Converse® high tops.

DERBIES
These are the ultimate guy shoes. Go for the classic, flower-toe models in thick leather, which is more masculine. The color should also be classic—black, navy, brown, camel, with an exception for metallic leather. A real pair of Church's or J.M. Weston's are a dream, but there are also beautiful models at Dr. Martens.

BOOTS AND ANKLE BOOTS
The same rules apply as for derbies. Go for the gorgeous dark-leather riding boots if your legs are long and slender; shorter options exist if need be. Avoid fancy embellishments at all costs, and choose thick soles that will help you gain a few precious centimeters. You can also venture into real ranger boots like the ones, again, at Dr. Martens.

12

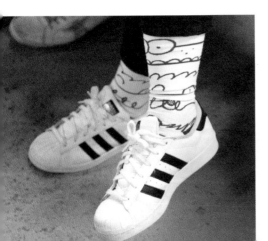

BALLET FLATS

These typically feminine shoes are lifesavers, so they shouldn't be overlooked. Personally I try not to wear them too often, because that would be taking the easy way out: "zero risk + comfort." You must wear them sparingly, or else you risk becoming an eternal teenager. Go for the classics like Repettos, unless you feel you can dare a pair of Marc by Marc Jacobs Mouse ballerina flats.

SANDALS

These are the exception to the rule of flats. Sandals rule in summer and all shapes are great, whether in simple leather at K-Jacques or Rondini or sprinkled with strass at Giuseppe Zanotti. Whether very mannish or super feminine, you'll never grow tired of them.

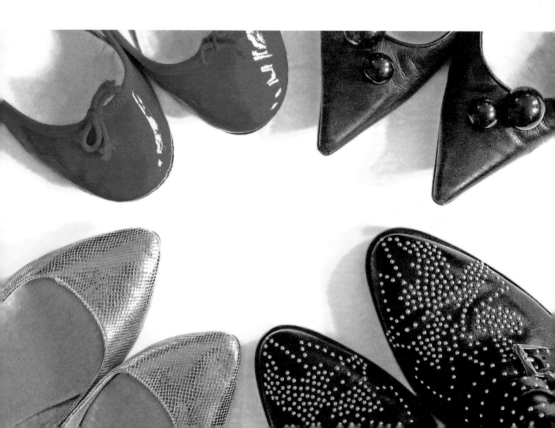

TAKE IT A **STEP FURTHER**

Now that all of this is clear, here are a few suggestions
to help show off your investment in your fine new slippers:

- Beautiful shoes are expensive so **take good care of them**.
A shoe repairman can superbly restore a rather worn-out pair, and finding a local shoe repairman can add decades to the life of your shoes.
- **Clean and polish** your shoes with quality products (like the Saphir brand for example).
- **Store them away** with care (*see* Day 5): maintain their shape with shoe trees and balled-up newspaper to keep the leather from creasing.
- **Pay special attention to your feet**. Though the feet wear the shoes, you often catch a glimpse of a rather average-looking foot spilling over the sides of luxury heels.

- Maintain a **good pedicure**.
- **Wear impeccable socks**, stockings, or pantyhose. Don't hesitate to play around with a look by adding a feminine touch to derbies paired with Swiss-dot stockings, or perking up very classic black heels with metallic silver anklets. Luxury is in the details, so have fun.
- **Be careful about the hems** of your pants; the wrong length can kill shoes. Don't hesitate to roll up your jeans to highlight your ankle and your high heels. Or break pleated pants onto the toes of very masculine derbies, which will compensate for their imposing look.

12

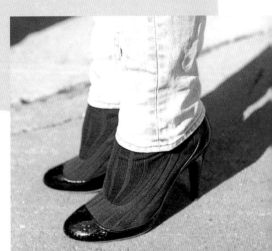

LET'S SEE YOUR SHOES TODAY!
#getgorgeous, #beautychallenge21

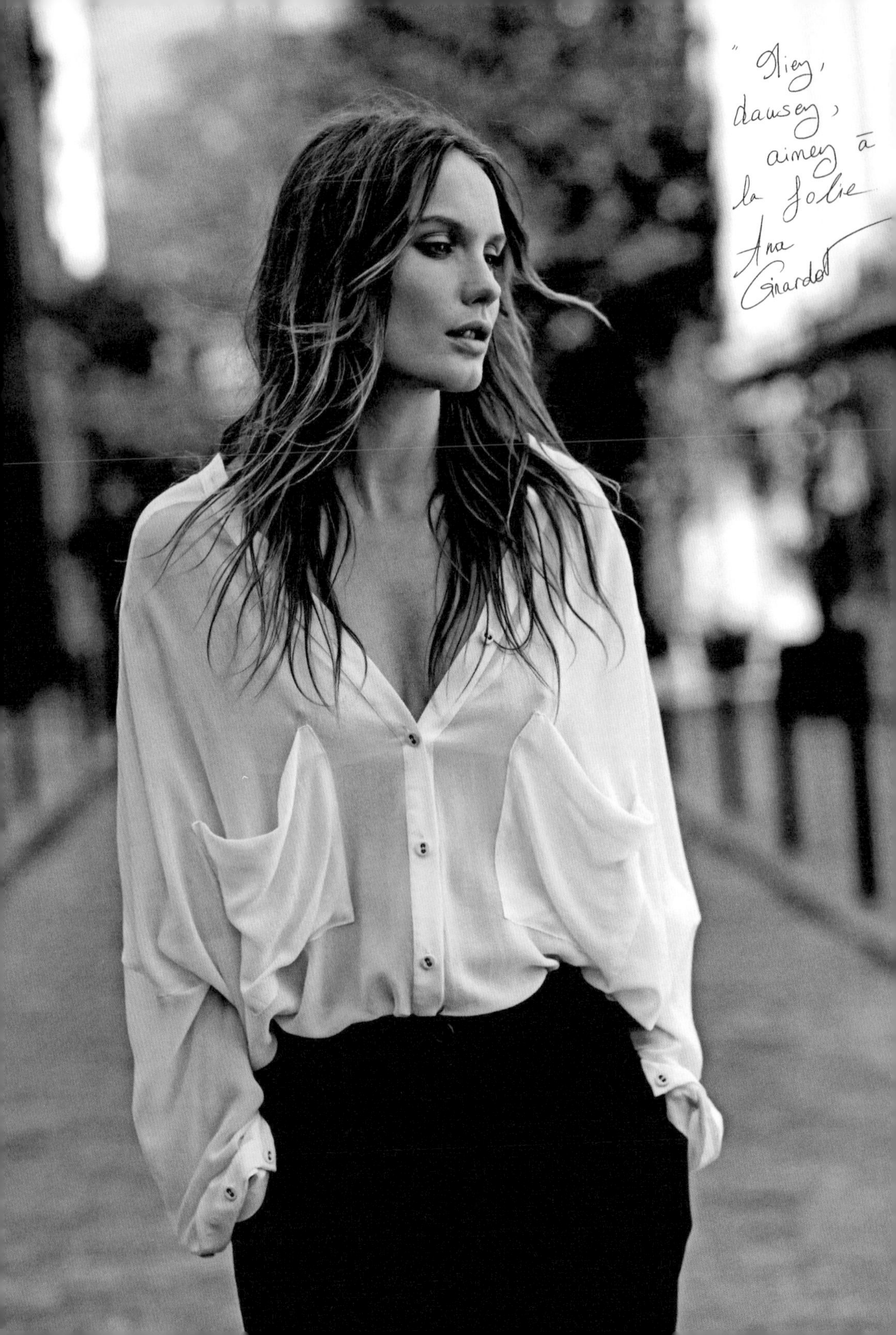
"Rier, danser, aimer à la folie
Ana Girardot

Ana Girardot

AGE: 27
PROFESSION: Actress
FIRST JOB: Babysitter
YOUR FAVORITE PHOTO OF YOURSELF: With my mother: we're laughing, we have the same smile
ASTROLOGICAL SIGN: Leo
DISTINGUISHING FEATURE: It's impossible for me not to smile
WHAT CAN'T YOU LIVE WITHOUT: Joy
WHAT DO YOU DO AS A SPECIAL TREAT FOR YOURSELF: Eat a huge breakfast
YOUR THREE SIGNATURE WARDROBE PIECES: Camel overcoat, Chanel bag, Saint Laurent heels
THREE MUST-HAVE BEAUTY PRODUCTS: Day cream, lip balm, mascara
YOUR PERFUME: It's a secret
WHO IS YOUR IDOL: Elvis
WHAT BOOK IS ON YOUR NIGHTSTAND: Stefan Zweig's *Twenty-Four Hours in the Life of a Woman*
YOUR LUCKY CHARM: My boyfriend
LESS OR MORE: Always more of less
YOUR MOTTO: "Every problem has a solution."
YOUR ADVICE FOR READERS: Live your life with passion, don't be afraid to scrape your knees.

Do you consider yourself a shoes addict?
I have way, way, way too many shoes.
High heels or flats? Mostly flats, but colorful.
How many pairs of shoes do you own? The photo says it all.
High heels—pleasure or pain? Pain! But what a look!
Your basic shoes: A pair of vintage Yves Saint Laurent kitten heels.
Your favorite designers: Chanel, Gucci, Topshop.
How do you take care of your shoes?
I don't really take care of them.... Guilty!
Do you have to spend a lot of money to have good shoes? Not necessarily, Zara has great shoes!
Your latest splurge: I am dreaming of Gucci's fur-lined slippers.... Is it too late?

———

Facing page: Laugh, dance, love passionately.

13

SELECTING MY

Accessories

EXTRAS ARE ESSENTIAL

ACCESSORIES
ARE A **MUST!**

"Details make perfection,
and perfection is not a detail."

Leonardo Da Vinci

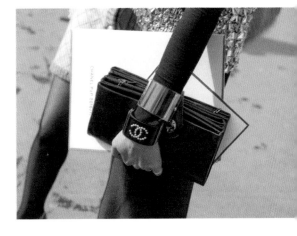

An accessory might seem like a detail, but it's key to the right look. It's what makes you chic and alluring. It's the little extra touch that transforms your outfit, the je ne sais quoi that makes all the difference. After all, "the devil is in the details."

Although it's true we strongly recommend that our models go to appointments dressed as simply as possible so the casting director can project without having to do an extreme makeover, we recognize that a good number of them have a knack for accessorizing, just like the stylists who dress them for photo shoots.

This is what makes their look unique when they come out of the fashion shows.

I've always loved accessories, from costume jewelry to totes, by way of scarves and glasses, **with the handbag being, for** **me, the ultimate accessory**. Yet—strangely paradoxical—I've always dreamed of being a man so I didn't have to carry one. How light it must feel to walk around with your hands in your pockets.

THE **LOWDOWN** ON **ACCESSORIES**

But before delving into the subject of handbags let's have fun reviewing accessories from head to toe, to get a better take on them.

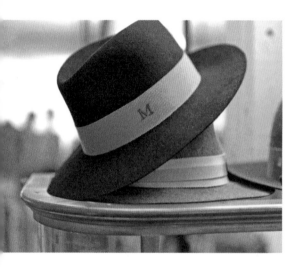

HATS

Initially this accessory was made to cover and protect the head. It may have been unthinkable to go out without one in the nineteenth and early twentieth centuries, but now we only wear one to enhance an outfit.
- Felt, originally used for a men's hats, creates a mysterious look.
- The American-style baseball cap makes you look like a teenager.
- The Gavroche cap is casual.
- Straw sun hats give you that Saint-Tropez appeal.
   Hats are the elegant touch that will give you panache.

KNIT CAPS

Essential when it's very cold, a knit cap can give your look style. Choose a solid color without embellishments. It will be chicer—after all, you're no longer a little girl.

CHINESE PORTRAIT

"IF I COULD COME BACK AS A FASHION ACCESSORY, IT WOULD BE A SHOPPING BAG."

KARL LAGERFELD

If I were a handbag, I would be:

....

If I were a pair of sunglasses, I would be:

....

If I were a hat, I would be:

....

If I were a scarf, I would be:

....

If I were earrings, I would be:

....

If I were a necklace, I would be:

....

If I were a bracelet, I would be:

....

If I were a watch, I would be:

....

If I were a men's accessory, I would be:

....

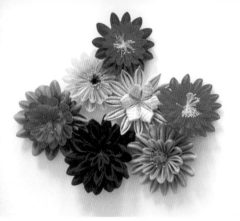

Hair Flowers by Karuna Balloo.

TIP

To downplay the nice-girl look of classics, wear just one earring and mix it with punk pieces, like a slim hoop and a metal stud.

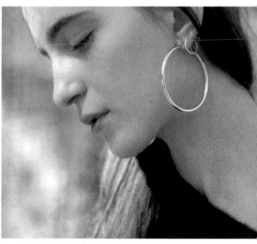

Fay - FORD MODELS.

HAIR ACCESSORIES

Headbands, bobby pins, barrettes, and flowers are there to make your hair look fabulous. They can give a romantic or an upbeat look to your hairstyle, but be careful not to overdo it. As usual when it comes to style, **less is more**!

EARRINGS

This is the accessory that lights up your face and embellishes it. When small brilliant stones appear behind a strand of hair, it's the ultimate in chic.

Women have been wearing jewelry since antiquity, and although for a long time our earlobes were only pierced with one or two holes, now the entire cartilage can be pierced.

Once again I recommend not overdoing it—three or four holes maximum—to avoid the hardware store look.

The past few years we have seen jewelry pieces that hug the shape of the entire ear. These rather impressive pieces should only be worn on one side and preferably with the hair pulled back to highlight the relevant ear.

You can be more conventional by wearing either a diamond brilliant in each ear, hoop earrings (either big or very small), or beautiful pearls. These great classics are a bit of an investment, but they are worth it because they're for a lifetime.

Stick to costume jewelry for bigger or more amusing pieces, like a long pendant or big rhinestone studs.

RINGS AND BRACELETS

These enhance our hands and our movements. We like just one single big ring on one hand, or simple slim bands on two or three fingers.

For some time now we've seen rings worn on the first or second phalanx, for offbeat elegance.

While creative costume rings do make an impact, it's preferable to invest in a ring of a certain value, like a signet ring that you wear on the pinkie for a chic, timeless look. Once your teenage years are behind you, investing in a beautiful ring is always a good idea.

Check out vintage and estate jewelry shops. You can get good bargains, notably with pieces from the 1930s, 1940s, and 1950s. For financial reasons, between World Wars I and II, and after World War II, beautiful synthetic stones were made, which were mounted on gold or platinum, making them more affordable.

Hang on to that precious, out-of-style ring your grandmother gave you. Go through all the little pieces of jewelry and gold that you own, and take them to a jeweler who will suggest salvaging the stones and metal to turn them into the piece you want.

The same goes for bracelets, which we sometimes forget about. Personally I like lots of colorful Bakelite bracelets or bangles, which are great for dressing up a simple cotton dress in summer, or lots of fine gold or silver bracelets—they make a little music with every flick of your wrist.

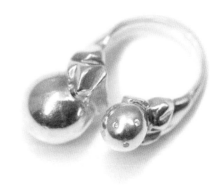

Ring by En Attendant Serge.

NECKLACES

Long *sautoirs,* collars, and chokers are today's bijou superstars. To brighten up your face and dress up your bust line, we like them long, mid-length, short, or fanciful. Remember that metal and stone are so many points of light that attract the eye and give you a vibrant look.

Every year I accompany my models to Cannes for the annual film festival. I love the moment when, after having chosen their red carpet gown, they are welcomed by top jewelers and adorned with diamonds.

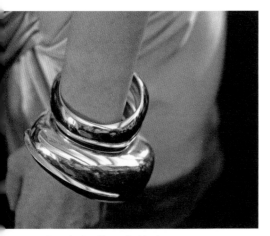

Bracelet by Alexandre Vauthier.

The models are used to this kind of thing, but the magic of gorgeous stones still works and I see their eyes light up. Basically we all have the soul of a princess.

Without spending a fortune, you can find slim gold chains and embellish them with small pendants that create a beautiful effect when put together. Accessories are made to be grouped; the simpler and more discreet they are, they easier it is to combine them to create a harmonious look, so go ahead and have fun.

BROOCHES

Originally these were worn near the heart, at chest level. But these pieces that our grand-mothers loved are now found on handbags or at the belt. Play around with them! A pretty brooch will highlight a basic sweater or a jacket that's too understated.

SUNGLASSES

These are obviously essential for protecting your eyes from harmful UV rays, but this is not their only quality. The glamorous touch of a mysterious look, or simply the best friend of a dull complexion and tired-looking eyes, the right pair of sunglasses is the hot item in the getting gorgeous process.

Sunglasses evoke movie stars. Go for it. Pretend you're from Hollywood. Wear them all the time, in winter or when it's gray out, and wear them extra large, with vintage,

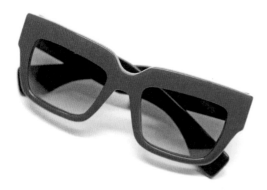

Prada sunglasses.

round, square, or butterfly frames. But be careful. I recommend trying several pairs at a good facialist optician, who will recommend what kind of frames to buy. There is nothing worse than glasses that don't suit the shape of your face.

Don't forget to clean your lenses before wearing them. It's a minor detail that makes all the difference.

Shopping tip: you can find great models from the 1950s–1970s in vintage shops.

FOULARDS

The scarves that used to protect us from drafts when we wrapped them around our neck are now popular for prettying up our wrists and handbag handles, and they're even used for belts. Choose noble materials like silk—I'm thinking of the famous Hermès Carré, their square silk scarf. I recommend wearing it over understated clothing to avoid a muddled look.

We often forget this, but a hanky, the scarf's second cousin, is an extremely feminine accessory. In silk, lace, chiffon, or very beautiful cotton, it is a very elegant detail.

Why not perfume it and negligently let it hang out of your handbag or jeans pocket. Or wear it like men do, in a blazer pocket.

Don't forget bandannas, the cult accessory of the 1980s. They are making a strong comeback and will be at their best tied in your hair in summer.

SCARVES AND WRAPS

These are wrapped around the neck and must be warm, in thick-knitted wool for a casual look, tartan for a posh effect, or cashmere jersey for luxuriousness. Oversized versions are preferable. Scarves should be fine but extra-long, wraps 40 × 40 inches (100 × 100 cm).

Styling tip: with long scarves, you can create good volume around your neck, which optically can create a slimmer look for the rest of your figure.

TIES AND BOWTIES

Borrowed from the men in our lives, these are ideal for an original, tomboy-style look.

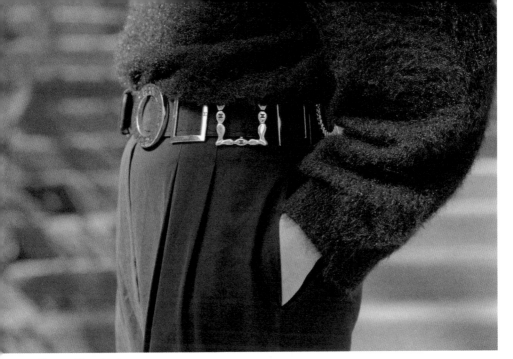

Vintage Chanel belt.

SUSPENDERS
These used to hold-up our trousers and now are worn on one shoulder only, for sexiness.

WATCHES
With our smartphones, we no longer need watches to tell the time. Yet it would be a shame to give up them up, since they can look like a bracelet. I'm not really a fan of showy models that are too new. Again, vintage is a safe bet. Simple shapes and understatement are always a guarantee of elegance: that's why men's models often create a better effect. Many jewelers today offer leather straps or colored canvas straps, a great trick for perking up a vintage model or the one you'll steal from your boyfriend. But don't forget the simple Swatch in colorful plastic, perfect for summer.

BELTS
Ideal for marking the waist and holding up our trousers, and also for making an outfit more fun. Again, be careful about cheap-looking belts: the great classic belt is made of leather, not fake leather! But canvas

is good too. Remember to choose belts that are a little long, then you can tie it at the end, for a more elegant look.

STOCKINGS AND SOCKS
Very visible when you wear shorts or a skirt, hardly at all when they peek out from a pant leg, these are basic accessories.

A pair of stockings can change the shape of your legs to make them look slenderer, or quite the opposite, cause them to look heavier.

Fishnet or Swiss dot stockings, couture stockings, and garter belts are incredibly seductive.

Colorful socks help give your look an infinite variety of new twists (*see* Day 16).

SHOES
There's so much to say about shoes, but we covered all the bases in the chapter dedicated to them (*see* Day 12).

HANDBAGS

"Never without my handbag!" A handbag is *the* accessory that all women absolutely have to have. You could write a book about them. Some have become cult items over time, like the Hermès Kelly bag and the Birkin. We put our entire life into our handbag. Whether big or small, classic or original, our bag is an extension of ourselves, so the subject merits close attention.

Remember to take care of it and polish it, not to just drop it down anywhere (have you seen those great portable hooks for hanging your bag from the edge of a restaurant or café table?), and don't overfill it, which will surely deform it.

There are so many handbags on the market that it is sometimes difficult to get your bearings. I can't tell you enough to stay away from "trendy" models. A beautiful bag is a major investment. So why buy a trendy one that, by definition, could go out of style quickly? Invest rather in more timeless shapes and models. Focus on leather quality. The leather has to be resistant and have a gorgeous patina. Be careful about materials that are too smooth, which can become very quickly scratched. Invest in classic colors like camel, black, navy, or Bordeaux. There are a number of ways to perk up a bag that's a little too understated for your taste:

- Tie a brightly colored foulard scarf to the handle.
- Hang a fun charm on it, like Prada's robot decorations or Fendi's little stuffed fur animals.
- Personalize it with your initials (many shoe repair shops offer this service).
- Accessorize the inside of your bag with small leather items in bright colors; this is where you can go with very trendy ones. For example, a coin purse, checkbook, address book, clutch, etc.

Finally, remember to regularly reorganize your handbag, and for the ultimate in perfection, spritz it with your favorite fragrance.

Styles are no longer minimalist, so don't hesitate to vary your accessories for a chic, offbeat, sparkly, or classic look. Now you have all the keys for choosing well. It's your turn to go out and play.

CLUTCHES AND MINAUDIÈRES

The perfect evening handbag. Because they are small, you can be a little imaginative and extravagant. Go for rhinestones, pick ones in precious fabrics (brocade, velvet, or silk), choose a rigid plastic or metal model, or even treat yourself to a wonderfully imaginative object like Olympia Le-Tan's book minaudières.

LET'S SEE YOUR FAVORITE HANDBAG.
\# #getgorgeous, #beautychallenge21

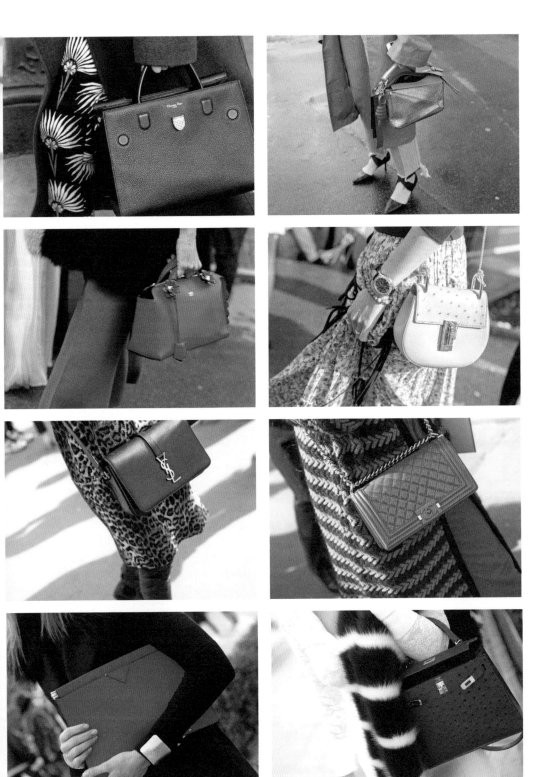

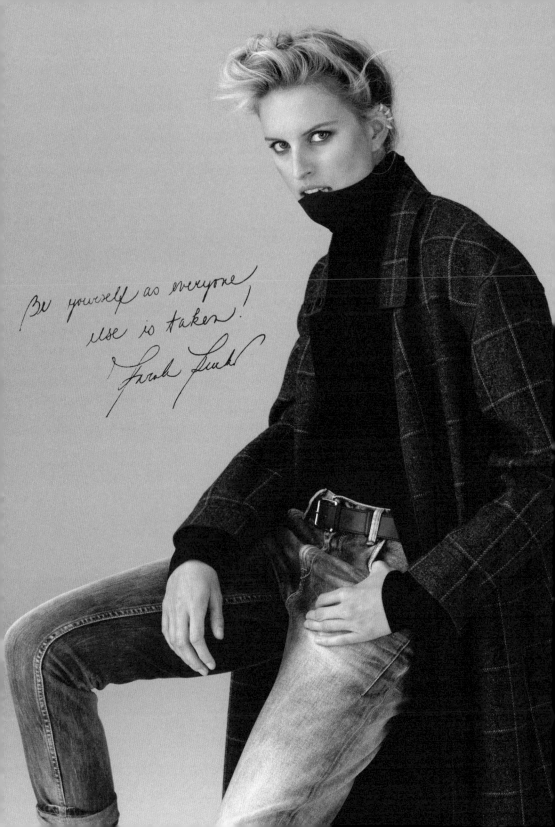

Be yourself as everyone,
else is taken!
Karolína Kurková

Karolína Kurková

AGE: 32
PROFESSION: Fashion model
FIRST JOB: My first big job was an exclusive contract with Prada and opening their show
YOUR FAVORITE PHOTO OF YOURSELF: Me as Marilyn Manson by Steven Meisel for *Vogue* with the help of the fantastic makeup artist Pat McGrath
ASTROLOGICAL SIGN: Pisces
DISTINGUISHING FEATURE: My legs and my laugh!
WHAT CAN'T YOU LIVE WITHOUT: Music and sunshine!
WHAT DO YOU DO AS A SPECIAL TREAT FOR YOURSELF: Body massage
YOUR THREE SIGNATURE WARDROBE PIECES: White button-down shirt, black blazer, white jeans
THREE MUST-HAVE BEAUTY PRODUCTS: Matte red lipstick, highlighter, eyebrow pencil
YOUR PERFUME: I use essential oils that I blend depending on my mood. One of my favorites is musk with little hint of something soft and delicate. I love when masculine meets feminine.
WHO IS YOUR IDOL: I admire so many people! The list would be too long!
WHAT BOOK IS ON YOUR NIGHTSTAND: *How Children Succeed* by Paul Tough
YOUR LUCKY CHARM: Don't have any, but I still feel lucky!
LESS OR MORE: Less AND more! Depending on the situation, the occasion, and my mood! I can definitely go both ways!
YOUR MOTTO: "Be yourself as everyone else is taken."
YOUR ADVICE FOR READERS: Always wear clothes you are comfortable with. Be inspired, don't give yourself a total look. Mix and match to follow your personality; don't be afraid, in the end feeling good is more important than what people think.

Can an outfit look good without many accessories? Yes, some clothes need nothing more than the right handbag and the right shoes.
Adding accessories can save your look: true or false? True! And a fun or beautiful accessory can even create the look and give it a twist. Always keep an eye open for details.
Should all your accessories match (bag, belt, shoes, etc.)? No, never!
Are you a minimalist who accessorizes with one statement piece, or a maximalist who adds layers of accessories to your look? It depends on the look I want to wear and what I am in the mood for. What I wear needs to match how I'm feeling and where I'm going.
Do you prefer novelty jewelry or investment pieces? Timeless accessories or seasonal, on-trend pieces? I like to have key timeless pieces that don't go out of style. They also have a sentimental value so I will keep them preciously. I'm very interested in the new designers emerging in magazines, exhibitions, concept stores. A piece of jewelry can make all the difference and there is a lot of creativity out there right now. So my advice: be curious.
Which must-have accessory is at the top of your wish list? I fall easily for a new pair of sunglasses! Along with handbags, they're always on top of my wish list! I can't live without a couple of earrings that follow me where ever I travel, they're easy to wear and make me feel like myself!

01
02
03
04
05
06
07
08
09
10
11
12
13
14
15
16
17
18
19
20
21

DAY

14

EASING INTO

Streetwear

WHERE COMFORT AND STYLE COEXIST

STREET STYLE

"I believe in comfort. If you don't feel comfortable in your clothes, it's hard to think about anything else."

Donna Karan

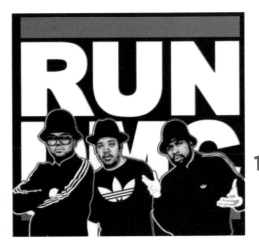

If to be well dressed and have style means to elegantly wear beautiful clothes (*see* Day 15), what about comfort? That feeling we get when we slip into cozy old flannel pajamas or sweatpants. Should we categorically refuse oversized shapes; wide, loose pants; and sneakers at all costs? No! We shouldn't. It all depends on the situation. And thanks to **streetwear**, which appeared in New York in the early 1970s, now we can be stylish and feel comfortable, too.

As the term streetwear suggests, the style comes from the street, and more precisely from the desire some people have to express their rebellion and rejection of society. The anarchistic statements of revolutionary youths constituted the basis of what became a style. Punks, skaters, and rappers all helped create this urban look, which the fashion industry soon spotted and democratized just as quickly.

In France, my generation remembers the "jeans + sweater" look of Vanessa Paradis in the video that made her famous, "Joe le Taxi"(1987). While first I had been drawn to those 1950s outfits, I quickly switched to the hip-hop look that went with the music I listened to. Like the rap groups I loved, I wore hoodies, leggings, and Adidas. In 1986, RUN-DMC, the famous 1980s rap group, dedicated a song, "My Adidas", to

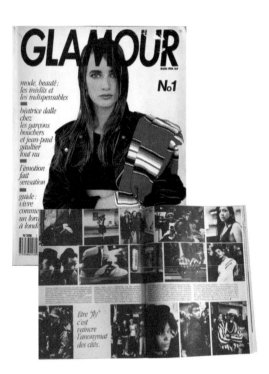

All of these labels offer a new take on streetwear basics, and since the 2000s they have called on music industry superstars to promote them. I remember running all over New York looking for the Bathing Ape shop that sold the famous hoodie worn by Pharell Williams!

That's when luxury brands started working with artists to create unusual, one-off collections, the famous "collaborations." Creating more buzz, it's a sales strategy that caused fashionistas to freak over "collector" editions often sold in concept stores. The biggest houses couldn't resist that kind of change, as the Chanel x Reebok InstaPump Fury sneaker that appeared in 2001 and the Junya Watanabe x Nike Vintage Running shoe that showed up in 2007 illustrate. For the biggest fans among us, there were limited edition collaborations like the Eminem x Jordan x Carhartt sneaker, among others.

Over the past few years, couture house and luxury ready-to-wear stylists have seized hold of streetwear. Givenchy designer Riccardo Tisci, who has always looked to urban culture to draw up his collections, has made no mistake in this. He has been working with Nike, for whom he designs the Nike x RT line, since 2014. Alexander Wang, too, has become a streetwear reference with his own brand. In 2012, he was unexpectedly named head of Balenciaga, which goes to prove the extent of the trend. The Italian house has just replaced him with Demna Gvasalia, founder of the Vêtements design collective, one of the Paris scene's latest "underground," edgy streetwear sensations. And props to Stella McCartney, who has worked with Adidas since 2004, nailing it with a line both technical and very feminine.

While I haven't invested in these brands' cool clothes or sneakers, I admit I fell for Isabel Marant's wedge sneakers—they're original and elegant.

the famous sneakers with three black bands on a white shoe.

The blueprint for that urban look was based on a few key elements: sweatshirts, wide jeans, "cycling" shorts, and huge sneakers. The women who adopted the look were called "Fly Girls"; the very first issue of French *Glamour* covered the style in 1988, echoing it in the fashion pages. This dress code, for a certain group of young people, changed a lot and became widespread initially due to the music, but above all because major brands like Adidas, Fila, Nike, and Carhartt, which have become classics today, had taken off. Kids who in the past wore the clothes from these stores, which were initially created to sell sports or work clothing, gradually witnessed the arrival of new streetwear brands like Rocawear and Ecko, and, in France, Wrung and Royal Wear. H&M and Zara put the final touch to the democratization of streetwear by selling every possible variation on it at affordable prices.

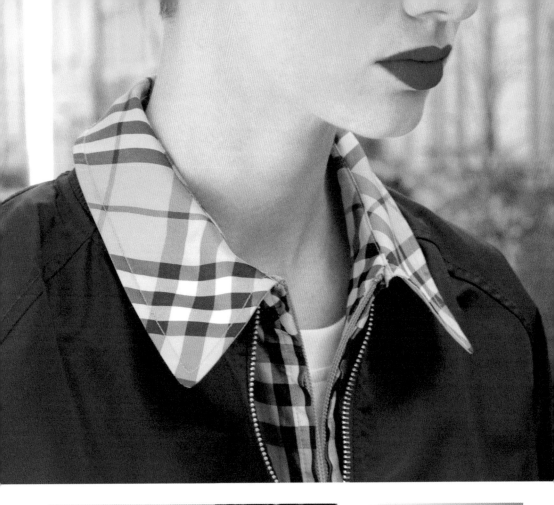
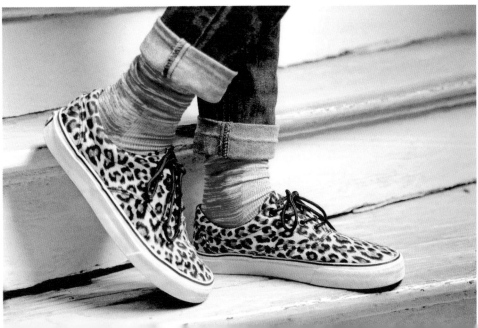

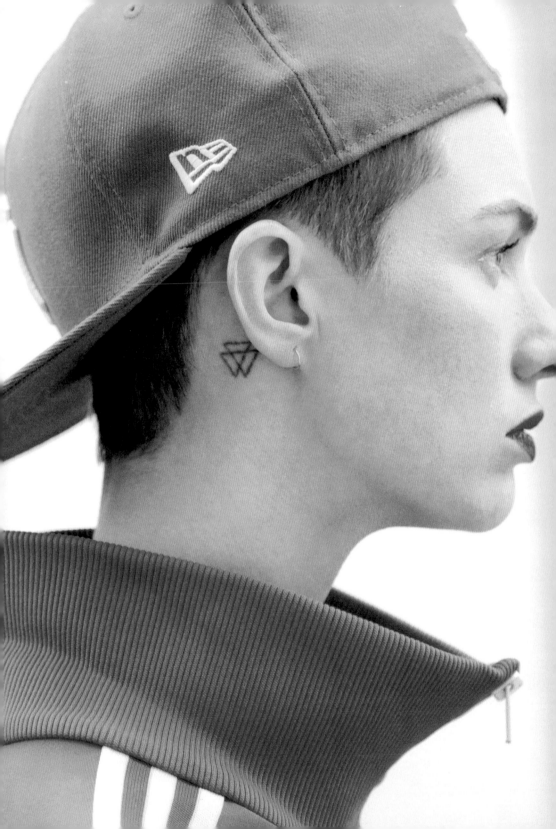

HOW DO YOU
WEAR STREETWEAR?

N ow that we've actually got some streetwear items in our closet, how can we wear them without looking like a high schooler? How, like models and stars who never leave home without their sneakers, can we give streetwear a newer, more elegant twist? Here are a few tricks for wearing basics such as caps, sweatshirts, sweatpants, and sneakers:

CAPS

Borrowed from baseball players and rap stars, caps can make any outfit look cool. Worn with a dress or any little ensemble, they'll give your look a modern, elegant touch. Choose a flashy color to perk up plain attire. Worn frontwards or backwards, a cap accents boyishness. If you have long hair, let it stick out from the cap. You can also tie your hair back in a ponytail or wear a braid over your shoulder. For mid-length hair, allow a few strands to fall around your face. If you have short hair, no prob. Just adjust your cap when you put it on—and voilà.

KNIT CAPS/BEANIES

Whether short and tight-fitting and with a cuff, or long for a softer look, and whether in winter wool or summer cotton, the beanie has become a key streetwear accessory. It saves my life on days when I'm clueless about what to do with my hair!

THE HOODIE

Is there anyone out there who has never worn a hoodie or crew neck sweatshirt? The kind

CAP STYLES

- **The Snapback:** A cap you can adjust at the back to fit any head size, simply by pressing the right snap.
- **The Strapback:** Resembles the Snapback, but a strap (often leather) serves to adjust it at the back.
- **The Trucker:** An American classic that often has a big but light piece of mesh fabric in the back.
- **The New Era:** From the legendary New Era brand, it's very fashionable at the moment, like other sports-fan caps. I recommend the soft visor for more style.

you used to wear only to the gym? Now it comes in short and long-sleeved versions from luxury brands (Versace, Moschino, Karl Lagerfeld). Personally I love the cushiness of sweatshirts, with or without pockets (often a kangaroo pouch): and you can wear them with slim pants or a miniskirt! I have them in all colors, with a preference for the ones with statements splashed across them. When I was head of the Ford Paris modeling agency, I developed a collaboration with Wrung and gave models sweatshirts with their first name printed on them. It was a big hit, and all our customers wanted one.

SWEATPANTS

Perfect for working out at home or playing sports, now you can wear them to work or for an evening out. But be careful, ONLY if you pair them with dressier pieces! Choose a model that's not too wide and combine it with a close-fitting top. We now find more stylized, figure-hugging sweatpants, which keeps them from looking baggy and shapeless. Wear them low at the waist and don't tighten the elastic belt too much. Also, choose them fitted at the ankle and preferably with a small hem. For a more feminine look, try them with high heels, which will prevent the overly casual look.

SNEAKER **BASICS**

- **Converse®:** The Chuck Taylor All Star is certainly the world's most famous canvas sneaker. From James Dean to Jane Birkin to Lady Gaga, everyone has owned a pair. Whether high top or low top, the white and the black are our favorites, but other colors are not bad either, especially to perk up neutral clothes.
- **Nike:** Choose the famous Air Max that you can customize on the Nike store website. Wear them with skinny jeans or a skirt to avoid looking too exercise-oriented.

- **Adidas:** The Stan Smith™ has that minimalist look we love, since it goes with everything and has unlimited combination possibilities. It works best with men's pleated pants.
- **Vans®:** Buy the iconic flat Authentic model. It's elegant, light, and worn more in summer with rolled-up pants (hipster style) or a pleated skirt. Whether it's the laceless slip-on or the classic model, at least you'll have a pair in your closet.

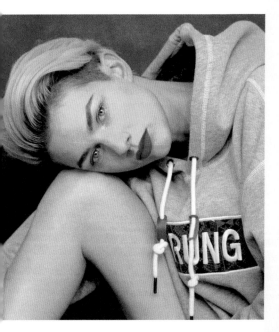

DON'T FORGET

- Espadrilles: we love to wear them on the seashore, and now in the city, too.
- Ugg Australia boots: totally comfortable and made famous notably by Sarah Jessica Parker in *Sex and the City*.
- Rivieras: a special shout out to the little Parisian brand that, over the past few years, has given us a new take on the grandpa-style slippers from southern Spain. In canvas or braided leather, they come in a wide range of fabulous colors for summer!

LEGGINGS

These long footless tights are to be worn in moderation. True, teenagers love them and they are very convenient. But their form-fitting fabrics can quickly give you pork legs, unless you look like a goddess!

SNEAKERS

These are perennial favorites, but for the past few years the fashion world hasn't been able to do without them. Sneakers are everywhere—worn by fashion editors and models and even spotted on catwalks. Though the classics are still in the forefront, there are now Chanel and Givenchy sneakers. They have to be worn in an unexpected way so you won't look like a Sunday jogger—for example, with a feminine dress or pretty pair of slacks—because it's the way they're put together that counts for a relaxed but well-dressed look. To keep it simple, I recommend the timeless basics and preferably in solid colors.

As you will have well realized, today we can combine our casual clothes with our classier pieces. This new trend called "athleisure"—a contraction of the words "athlete" and "leisure"—is a new way of dressing in sports clothes and shoes for urban activities. An increased awareness of overall wellness, and the revival or expansion of practices such as yoga, Pilates, and jogging have boosted the popularity of sports brands, which are now creating clothes with more style and design savvy. It is now "trendy" to show that you're athletic and to combine your sports clothes with your city basics. Follow the example of today's stars and don't hesitate to go out in streetwear or "athleisure" clothes.

WHO HAS THE BEST SNEAKERS? POST YOUR FAVORITE PAIR!

#getgorgeous, #beautychallenge21

Restez vous-même en
toute circonstance
Noémie Lenoir

Noémie Lenoir

AGE: 36
PROFESSION: Model
FIRST JOB: Dogsitter
YOUR FAVORITE PHOTO OF YOURSELF:
A cover by Mario Testino for French *Vogue*
ASTROLOGICAL SIGN: Virgo
DISTINGUISHING FEATURE: A beauty
mark between the eyes
WHAT CAN'T YOU LIVE WITHOUT: My children
WHAT DO YOU DO AS A SPECIAL TREAT
FOR YOURSELF: Go to the movies
YOUR THREE SIGNATURE WARDROBE PIECES:
A pair of heels, leather pants, a solid T-shirt
THREE MUST-HAVE BEAUTY PRODUCTS: Moisturizing
cream, sunscreen, and a bottle of spray mist
YOUR PERFUME: Tom Ford's White Suede
WHO IS YOUR IDOL: Mother Theresa
WHAT BOOK IS ON YOUR NIGHTSTAND:
Cyrano de Bergerac by Edmond Rostand and
Célibataire longue durée (longterm single)
by Véronique Poulain
YOUR LUCKY CHARM: A seashell, a gift from my son
LESS OR MORE: Less hatefulness, more respect
YOUR MOTTO: "Do not judge me by my
successes, judge me by how many times
I fell down and got back up again."
YOUR ADVICE FOR READERS (facing page):
Be yourself in all situations.

Is it a mistake to wear street style because it's more comfortable? No. It's very important to feel at ease and comfortable in your clothes when you know you're going to spend the day in them.
Is it possible to mix streetwear with more sophisticated pieces? Of course. Jeans and beautiful sneakers with a shirt or a hip jacket, for example; the possibilities are endless. Personally, if I have an important meeting, a reception, or a wedding, I prefer something chic like a dress. If I wear jeans, I wear a beautiful jacket and heels, paired with couture accessories.
Are sneakers anti-feminine? No, but it depends on the pair. I would never wear Jordans with a skirt, I'm too old for that now. But a pair of Stan Smith™ sneakers, for example, with well-cut pants and a sexy, elegant T-shirt can be very feminine.
Can a red-carpet look be comfortable? It's an honor to wear sumptuous dresses. And when I feel beautiful, I feel at ease. I could even wear a corset.
What are your tricks for not suffering in heels? Twenty years of modeling make the feet. If the arch of the shoe and the heel don't suit me, I change the pair or brand (arches differ with brands).
What designer does the best job of pairing street style with comfort? Riccardo Tisci at Givenchy.

01
02
03
04
05
06
07
08
09
10
11
12
13
14
15
16
17
18
19
20
21

DAY

15

Styling

MY LOOK

MAKE IT MY OWN

WHAT DOES IT MEAN TO HAVE **STYLE**?

"Fashions fade, style is eternal."

Yves Saint Laurent

S tyle, that little something extra. Some women have effortless style. Elegance, an aura, a look—style is that visual identity that is so difficult to define because it varies from person to person.

As I write these words, an ad featuring Iris Apfel, the famous New York fashion icon who is now 94 years old, keeps showing in a loop on TV. Her motto: "I don't have any rules as I would always be breaking them so it would be a waste of time.... No trends, no rules, but I have style."

At a time when much emphasis is placed on images of oneself, standing out has become a real challenge. Not being like others, or being noticed because of your look and bearing is for some women the ultimate aim, as we observe in the colorful outfits of stylists such as Anna Dello Russo, or in the rather particular hairstyle of Anna Wintour.

Standing out from others, including from people in a group with the same references, and showing yourself to be different because of your clothes, voice, and gait are all ways of having style.

Possessing a certain assurance and wonderful self-image is not something we are born with, and it takes years for a style to take shape. Having style, or what younger people call "swag," is to find in yourself the feature, if not the flaw, that you are going to highlight so that you stand out. Rossy De Palma, for example, turned her rather large nose into her hallmark.

Style is timeless and it's why we continue to admire the classiness of Audrey Hepburn, for whom "elegance is the only beauty that never fades." It's why we like Grace Jones's look and Madonna's eccentricity.

A touch of Paloma-Picasso-style red lipstick, a hat tipped like Anna Piaggi's, a T-shirt worn simply, like Jane Birkin's, are strong, recognizable symbols of identity that we immediately associate with these icons.

HOW DO YOU ACQUIRE **STYLE**?

I don't know if there is a magic recipe, but here are a few rules to help you gain a sense of style!

• Cultivate a certain kind of **uniqueness** and have **self-confidence**. Be sure of yourself.

• Stake a **claim** to **elements of fashion,** but not just in any old way. It's no use spending a fortune, just pick the colors and shapes that make you beautiful and wear them. You now know your morphology (*see* Day 1). A little trick if you want to know what looks good on you is to trust other people's reactions. If when you wear a pair of slim jeans you get a lot of great compliments, go for this type of pants.

• Be **curious**. Look, dig around, get inspiration from fashion icons, magazines, the women around you.

• Get **personal**. Above all, do not seek to please everyone.

• **Repeat**. Wearing the same clothes or the same outfit repeatedly over time will help you create a strong identity. Having style is a matter of sending out a clear message. Watch designers like Karl Lagerfeld: they give the impression that they are always dressed in

the same way. You can well imagine that it's not due to lack of money or inspiration. It's simply due to great self-awareness and the desire to create a vision of themselves that will transcend fashions and times. This is the uniform we talked about (*see* Day 10).

• **Wear what looks good** on you, regardless of trends.

• **Be real**. Be genuine and give in to pleasure. There is nothing worse than wearing clothes you don't feel good in, just because you think they're fashionable.

• **Don't conform**. Stick to your guns.

• **Don't succumb** to influence. Listen to your body. Wear clothes suited to your morphology. Clothes worn by a model who is 6 feet tall (1 m 80) won't necessarily look good on a women who is 5 foot 2 inches (1 m 50). Each and every one of us has made the mistake—the memorable blunder—of letting ourselves be influenced by the dictates of fashion.

• **Don't try to stand out at all costs**. Having style does not mean being eccentric. Too much originality kills style, as we can observe when, after the fashion shows are over, out

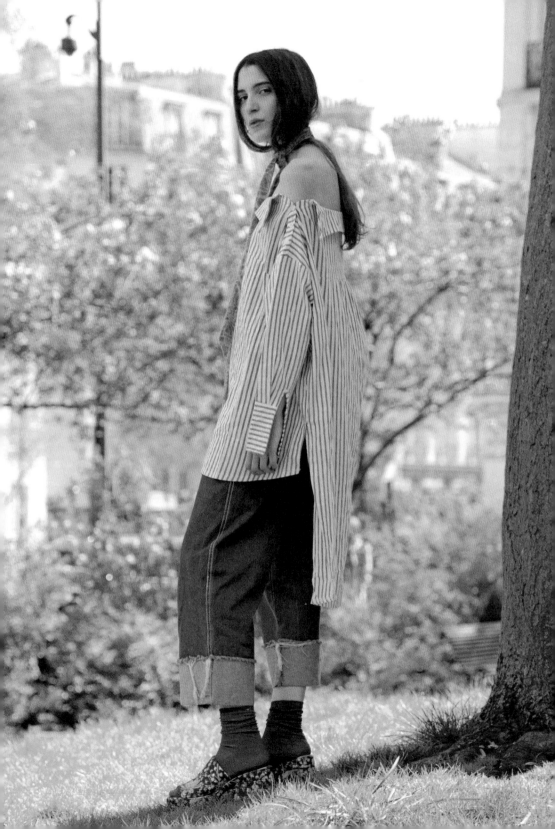

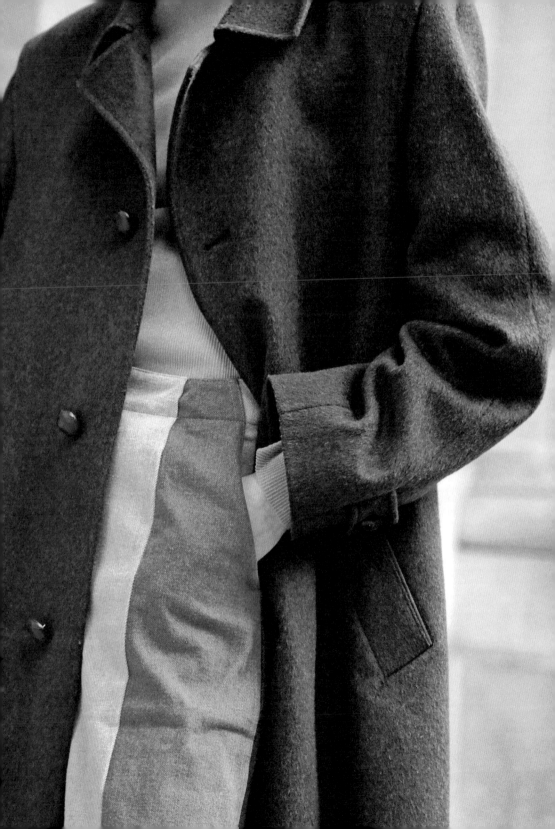

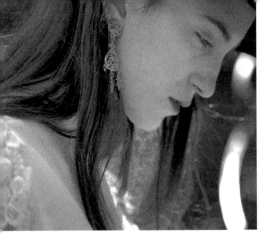

to keep quiet at public appearances. Her absolute silence left no one indifferent, encouraging people's imagination to run wild.

• Finally, **BELIEVE IN YOURSELF**. It's a simple trick of personal development. Even if you are plagued by self-doubt, learn to love yourself, to value your worth, to compliment yourself. After all, why should everyone else think you have style if you are not 100% convinced of it? For that, take a minute to stand in front of your mirror every morning and say to yourself, "I am beautiful and elegant and I like my style."

come the fashionistas, who can at times look ridiculous trying to get noticed by wearing outlandish clothes.

• **Make an effort** with your appearance. Clean, well-ironed clothes make all the difference.

• **Work on your bearing**. Having style means having charm. By the same token, pay attention to your gait. Style is elegance. This is one of the things I learned from top models. They are all able to move around with grace, sometimes slowly, and to stand straight, to occupy a room as though they were the only person in it. Yoga and ballet are excellent exercises for developing good posture and bearing.

• **Pay attention to your voice and how you speak**. Certain voices are a style in and of themselves—I am thinking of the low, hoarse quality of Jeanne Moreau's or Demi Moore's voice. Expressing yourself firmly and with determination yet with poise will give you a certain aplomb. Silence is also a good weapon at times. Mysterious people are always attractive. Marie-Françoise Santucci did a very good job of reading into the famously mysterious Kate Moss in her biography of the supermodel. The answer is simple: she started to fascinate crowds once she understood how important it was

WHAT STYLE IS NOT

In our society governed by immediacy, fashion victims' consumerism, and short-lived glory, having style is not a question of following trends at any price, but rather finding what looks good on you and you alone. Of course when we talk about style, we also talk about categories of looks, like a punk or preppy look. Stylists and photographers love this for titles of fashion series. These clothing styles are not "the" style.

15

CHRISTEL'S **TIPS**

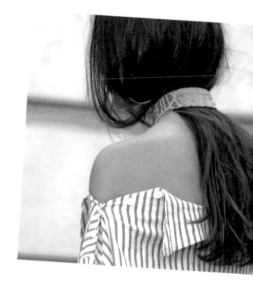

Did you know that at fashion shows, brands surround themselves with influential magazine stylists to help designers "style" their collection? It is always surprising to see how much influence their work can have on the presentation of a collection. Small details can really change how clothing is perceived. Details abound, and in spite of my experience with them, I must admit that I am always discovering new ones.

One of the best ways to learn about them is to watch people you come across and who you find well dressed, or else to scrutinize the "street style" pages in women's magazines.

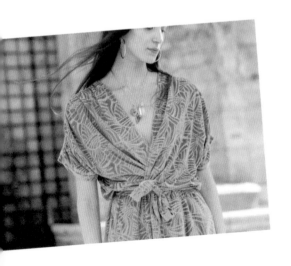

Reveal

A shoulder when you wear an oversized top.

Belt it

Your dresses, your coats.

Roll up

Your shirtsleeves, your jacket sleeves. Not to mention your jeans and pants.

Borrow

Your boyfriend's famous white shirt, big watch, or sweater, but perk it up with a narrow belt.

Mix and match

Shapes, fabrics, and lengths. A clingy T-shirt with a puffy miniskirt.

Wear

A coat or blazer over your shoulders (without slipping your arms into the sleeves).

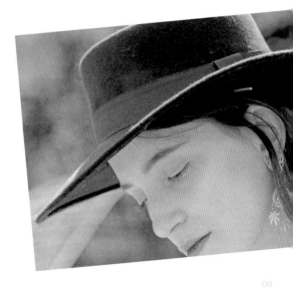

Accessorize

A gorgeous brooch on a coat.
Just one, but very big, earring.
A vintage handbag with a classic look.
A great-looking hat.

Skip

The shoelaces on your derbies.

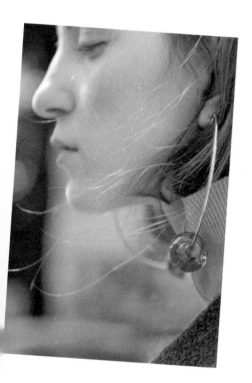

Pull out

Your shirttail—tug it out from your pants a bit (to avoid the "neatly tucked in" look).

WHAT IS YOUR WINNING STYLE TIP? SHARE IT!
#getgorgeous, #beautychallenge21

08
09
10
11
12
13
14
15
16
17
18
19
20
21

177

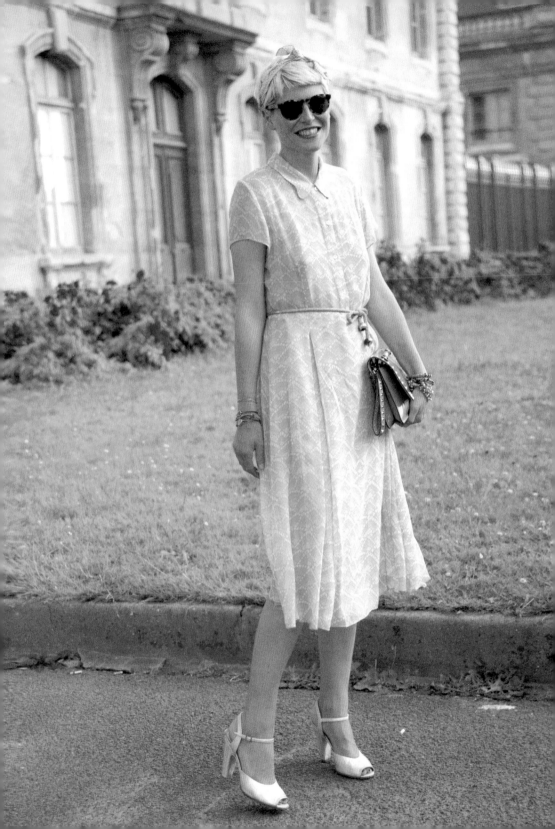

Elisa Nalin

AGE: 38
PROFESSION: Stylist, consultant, mother
FIRST JOB: Junior designer at Costume National
YOUR FAVORITE PHOTO OF YOURSELF: The pictures I like have one thing in common: my smile!
ASTROLOGICAL SIGN: Pisces, ascendant Taurus
DISTINGUISHING FEATURE: Almost always smiling
WHAT CAN'T YOU LIVE WITHOUT: Humor
WHAT DO YOU DO AS A SPECIAL TREAT FOR YOURSELF: Two hours of traditional Thai massage
YOUR THREE SIGNATURE WARDROBE PIECES: A sky blue silk men's shirt, a masculine pair of navy blue straight-cut slightly cropped trousers, a pair of slip-on Mira Mikati sneakers
THREE MUST-HAVE BEAUTY PRODUCTS: Black mascara, matte red lipstick from M·A·C, Dior Glow Maximizer Light Boosting Primer for a radiant face
YOUR PERFUME: Ginger eau de parfum by Centrale Formentera that I discovered in a little perfume shop in San Francisco on Formentera island
WHO IS YOUR IDOL: I wouldn't use the term idol; I admire Coco Chanel, Wallis Simpson, and my grandmother
WHAT BOOK IS ON YOUR NIGHTSTAND: At the moment, it's my friend Betony Vernon's *Boudoir Bible*
YOUR LUCKY CHARM: My 1,000 souvenir travel bracelets that I always wear on my left wrist
LESS OR MORE: More, of course
YOUR MOTTO: "Always be responsible for your actions, words, and thoughts. No one and nothing else is responsible for what happens in your life. Always search from within, not outside of yourself."
YOUR ADVICE FOR READERS: Be yourself; don't be afraid to take some risks, laugh more, start using more colors in your life and your wardrobe.

A single look or several styles? My style is eclectic and changes often: one day I'll feel like a tomboy and the next day ultra-feminine in a vintage '40s floral print dress, but—through accessories, my hairstyle, colors—my style will remain recognizable overall. I've always had my own style. As a little girl growing up in a small town like Verona, everyone dressed and looked the same; the only thing I wanted was to be different from the other girls. From a very young age, I was passionate about clothes, shoes, and fashion. It's important for me to stay authentic—without emulating anyone else—and to follow my unique personal taste.
Should we follow trends? In our hyper-connected world, we are constantly influenced by what we see around us. I don't follow trends; I'd rather create my own. But I have a sense for what's timely, and draw on it when creating my outfits.
What are your top three style tips? 1. Mix styles, prints, and colors. Polka dots with stripes, floral prints with plaid. 2. Break the rules. 3. Never be afraid to go overboard, but remember that it has to be worn by a real woman, in the real world. I only approve looks that I would wear personally.
Can styling change a garment's look? Absolutely! How you wear a garment can radically change its allure. There are a thousand different ways to wear a men's shirt, based on how it's combined with the rest of the outfit, accessorized, how we style our hair. All it takes is a little imagination.
Do you think it's possible to cultivate an aura? Yes, absolutely. Cultivate your inner self! Take care of your soul and cultivate spirituality. Keep digging; go beyond the surface. I'm convinced that inner beauty shows on your face, and increasingly so with age.

DAY

16

GIVING IT A

Twist

ADD SOMETHING QUIRKY

DESIGNERS, SOURCES OF **INSPIRATION**

To give a twist to your look
is to add an original touch to a basic look.

Applied to fashion, the idea is to perk up a look by adding a detail, or an unexpected, miscast accessory, to create an edgy look, one that makes a clean break from looking too proper.

This is the great specialty of English designers, who never hesitate to provoke and amuse you by giving new meaning to clothes and accessories. Of course Vivienne Westwood and Paul Smith come to mind, as does the brilliant Loewe designer Jonathan Anderson in a certain way. I remember running into Paul Smith many times backstage at his shows. What always struck me, in addition to his kindness, was that he seemed like a big kid, one who was always ready to crack jokes with his models; in contrast to most designers who are very distant, if not completely stressed out, on the day of their show.

Although he's American, it's impossible not to mention the wild troublemaker Jeremy Scott in this category. He made an impact with streetwear filled with Pop influences and is terribly successful today as head of Moschino, where he delivers collections known for being witty and eccentric, inspired by McDonald's and Coca-Cola packaging, for example, and by cartoon heroes.

These designers have a mutual love of color, keen sense of accessorizing, and ability to surprise by using humorous references. They can take a step back from the sometimes overly serious fashion world. Obviously, it's big business we're talking about, and the stakes and pressure are high; but we mustn't forget that fashion has to cultivate lightness and humor so it won't become gloomy or intimidating.

France has its own breed of designers who have cultivated eccentricity and kept a certain distance throughout their career. There's Jean Charles de Castelbajac and his famous Teddy Bear coat, made with stuffed animals and worn by pop stars (Madonna, Diana Ross). And there's Sonia Rykiel. This Saint-Germain-des-Prés icon could have

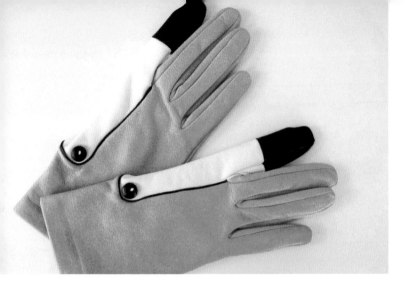

Gloves by Yaz Bukey.

taken an easy out and offered very classic bourgeois looks, but she always knew that wasn't enough. By always keeping a fun note in her collections—where you regularly find disco references that could be considered tacky, but that go so well with her little knit outfits—she came up with a recipe that still works today. For Sonia Rykiel, color is key—just think of all those multicolored stripes—and so are cheerfulness and joviality. Backstage at her shows, models are specifically asked to smile on the catwalk, in contrast to what is done everywhere else.

To me, it's the Italians who are the subtlest masters of giving fashion a twist. Miuccia Prada is certainly the queen of it. Unquestionably elegant, and a creative genius, she has that incredible knack of reinventing herself every season while staying on course for a very personal, recognizable style. She meets the challenge of creating shapes not devoid of classic touches, using clearly luxurious fabrics that are always rather witty and filled with offbeat references. I am thinking of her very colorful geometric prints here, her nutty accessories—the bags and shoes with a look very much inspired by 1950s American cars—or her multicolor rabbit prints.

Stylists for Italian magazines, like Anna Piaggi, the legendary and dearly departed editor in chief of *Vogue Italia* and Anna Dello Russo, creative consultant for *Vogue Japan*, were never afraid to surprise, if not shock you, by sitting in the front row at fashion shows and sporting outfits practically meant to look like disguises or theater costumes.

As you can well imagine, it's important to have fun with your look, to break the rules, give things a tasteful twist. It shows that you have personality and, quite simply, that you have a zest for life and know how to please yourself!

Obviously it's not about becoming a clown and rushing to buy the first fun or colorful accessory you come across. In this rather subtle, but fascinating exercise, you must remember that you don't want to look "amusing," but simply beautiful, radiant, and different.

"I'M ATTRACTED TO PEOPLE WHO MAKE THIS EFFORT IN KNOWING WHAT SUITS THEM— THEY ARE INDIVIDUAL AND STYLISH."

VIVIENNE WESTWOOD

A FEW
RULES

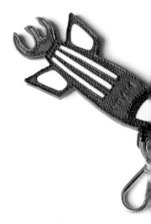

Prada keychain.

1 USE **COLOR**

Color is one of the major criteria, along with shape, that will guide you along when you buy clothes. As we explained earlier (*see* Day 4 and Day 5), it is important to know your colors, the colors that flatter you. For the sake of efficiency, it's preferable to work with two or three basics (black, gray, navy, white, indigo blue, camel) rather than to keep buying clothes without any sense of where you're headed. Then again there is nothing to keep you from perking up a monochrome look or a subtle range of colors with a lively, unexpected burst of color—and it's highly recommended. As often in fashion, less is more, and a detail can perk up an entire look, so limit yourself to using one bright color that will strengthen its impact. The possibilities for combining colors are numerous. It would take too long to cite them all, but you can try blood red with khaki, Indian rose with navy, fluorescent yellow and pale gray, or mix teal with flesh tones.

2 COMBINE **TEXTURES**

Another variable that can perk up a look is texture. Playing on the organic aspect of clothing is an excellent alternative if you don't want to use color. You can give a twist to a totally black look by contrasting knits and leather, matte and shiny materials, or very smooth fabrics with those with a bit of relief. Little moiré touches can also prove to be very interesting, whether it's a pair of shoes or a metallic leather handbag, a bijou, beautiful zipper, or buttons.

3 CONTRAST **SHAPES**

When it comes to fashion, you shouldn't hesitate to combine extremes. You can soften a tightly fitted look with a clearly oversized sweater, or, on the contrary, wear wide pants with a tight turtleneck, which will pep up the whole outfit. A long men's shirt is great with short jean shorts; and very long pants with a sexy crop top is also the ticket. Offsetting small and large sizes creates a sort of visual "surprise" and while you're at it, helps you hide certain flaws in your morphology.

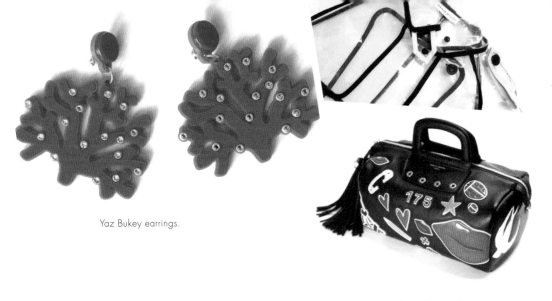

Yaz Bukey earrings.

Wanda Nylon trench coat.
Sonia Rykiel handbag.

GO WILD

Animal prints (leopard, zebra, and even snakeskin) are often pointed out as symbols of bad taste, but don't fall for this line, as it is absolutely false. Just look at any number of photographs of Carine Roitfeld and you'll understand they can be used with great elegance. So don't stop yourself from combining a pair of leopard stilettos with a total camel look or wearing that snakeskin-print leather jacket with jeans and a white T-shirt: perfect!

4 DARE TO COMBINE DIFFERENT PRINTS

Who ever said you couldn't mix polka dots and plaid, or mix a Glen plaid Prince of Wales check with stripes? People able to harmoniously blend the most daring patterns are fascinating. The golden rule is to mix only similar colors. Have fun combining navy-blue pinstripe men's pants with a white shirt with navy polka dots. If you're new at this, limit yourself to combining two different prints and add one large solid piece in the same color to unify the look.

5 BET ON ACCESSORIES

Using and even abusing accessories (*see* Day 13) is certainly the simplest, funnest, and certainly most economical way to give your look a twist.

Try giving your look a spark of quirkiness, take your time, find just the right dose, and, above all, enjoy yourself. Believe me, you won't regret it.

WHO HAS THE BEST ACCESSORY? LET'S SEE IT!
\# #getgorgeous, #beautychallenge21

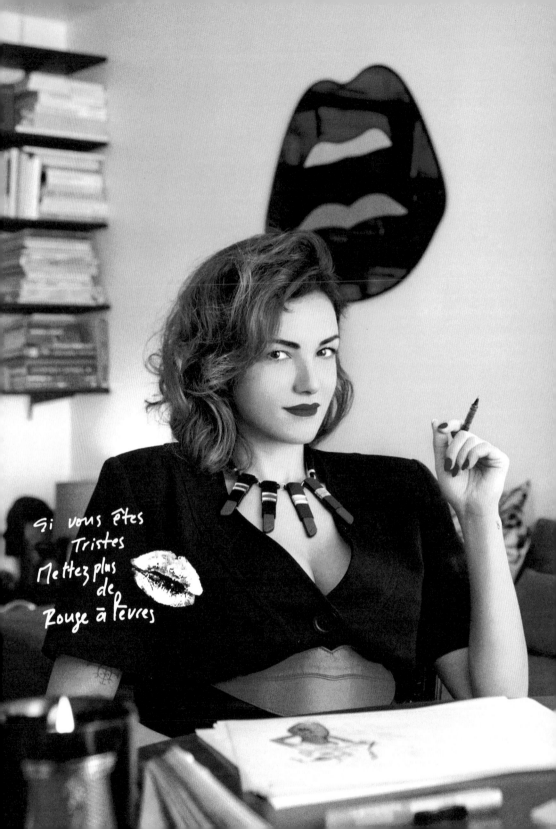

Si vous êtes
Tristes
Mettez plus
de
Rouge à lèvres

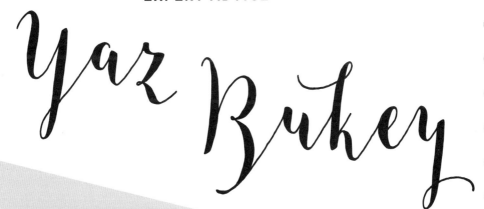

Yaz Bukey

AGE: Forever 16!
PROFESSION: "Sophisti-pop" designer
FIRST JOB: Radio announcer for the
Mickey Mouse Club, at the age of 12
YOUR FAVORITE PHOTO OF YOURSELF:
My portraits by the photography duo
Tania et Vincent
ASTROLOGICAL SIGN: Part Leo, part Virgo;
I was born on the 23rd, so depending on
the astrologer, it's one or the other
DISTINGUISHING FEATURE: Total insomniac
WHAT CAN'T YOU LIVE WITHOUT:
Meditation and exercise
WHAT DO YOU DO AS A SPECIAL TREAT FOR
YOURSELF: Drink a cocktail at the pool
YOUR THREE SIGNATURE WARDROBE PIECES: My
Hervé Leroux and Azzedine Alaïa dress collections
and my collection of heels (350 pairs and counting)
THREE MUST-HAVE BEAUTY PRODUCTS: My
red lipstick—Sue Uemura's Yaz Red, Erborian's
BB cream, and Shiseido's powder compact
YOUR PERFUME: Byredo's M/Mink
WHO IS YOUR IDOL: My aunt,
Princess Fawzia of Egypt
WHAT BOOK IS ON YOUR NIGHTSTAND:
I prefer reading into images!
YOUR LUCKY CHARM: Viktor, my
Chihuahua Miniature Pinscher
LESS OR MORE: Why less when
you can have more?!
YOUR MOTTO: "Indestructible!" One day when Cher
was asked what would remain if the planet were
destroyed by a nuclear bomb, she replied: "Cher
and the cockroaches." We have the same motto!
YOUR ADVICE FOR READERS (facing page):
If you feel sad, put on more lipstick!

**Do you agree with Friedrich Nietzsche that "The
devil is in the details"?** Yes, but don't sweat it!
**Fashion is serious business—does that exclude
humor in design?** These days, especially, we need
more time and freedom as creative people. After
that, either you have a sense of humor or you don't.
What made you want to start creating accessories?
I wanted accessories (I hate this word) to take
over the clothing. For me the clothes are the
showcase for the accessories. In addition, I've
been working for some time on the idea of the
personal accessory and the home accessory.
**Do you remember the first accessory you ever
created?** A fox mask strewn with pearls.
It is important to be daring? You have to express
yourself. I need to mix pieces and express my
mood of the day, but I don't feel the need to
explain it, just to send out a message. The look is
an overall statement! From head to toe, including
hairstyle, makeup, accessories, and heels.
Whay clothing detail always attracts your eye?
Shoes. Show me your shoes, I'll tell you who you are!
What colors perk up a look?
The colors of the rainbow!
An accessory you're crazy about?
My cigarette holder.
**Lipstick is a recurring theme for you—do you
have other beauty obsessions?** Fake lashes!
You would never go out without…?
An impeccable manicure.

DAY

17

GETTING

Picture Perfect

WHAT IS THE SECRET TO A GREAT SELFIE?

SAY **CHEESE**

"Selfie: a photograph that one has taken of oneself,
typically one taken with a smartphone
or webcam and shared via social media."

Oxford Dictionary

Taking selfies has become very trendy over the last few years. In the past we were beholden to others when having our snapshot taken. Smartphones and other technological tools freed us up from that. The selfie is everywhere now. It is the prerogative of teenagers and stars, who share their portraits widely through social media. It can seem like the height of narcissism, and it's a trend that has many detractors. Yet in an era where images predominate, what could be better than controlling yours? Self-portraits have been around for ages; why not make the most of them?

Learning to love yourself comes through your self-image, and without going deep into the psychology of it, wanting to show yourself in the best light is entirely natural. Besides, if some women hate seeing themselves in photos, it's often due to a lack of self-confidence. No longer averting your eyes from your own image, and actually looking at yourself is often a first step towards self-acceptance. The selfie can turn out to be excellent therapy for learning to love yourself.

From childhood on, we are photographed for a diverse variety of reasons, whether for ID cards, class pictures, photos that forever capture on film wonderful summer memories, and photos of countless other moments that we have long since forgotten.

Personally, I have never minded being photographed, but on one condition—being in top form—and the same goes for photos of others, too.

An Indian proverb comes back to me every time I find myself behind or in front of a camera: "when you take someone's picture, you steal their soul." If this is true, I think we should always photograph the people around us with the greatest generosity and lots of love. Showing them to their best advantage and even glorifying them seems the least we can do. It's part of my philosophy of life: to always see things—and people—in the best light.

So, whether you are the camera's subject or the person who presses the button, be sure to put your best foot forward.

17

IN **SELFIE** MODE

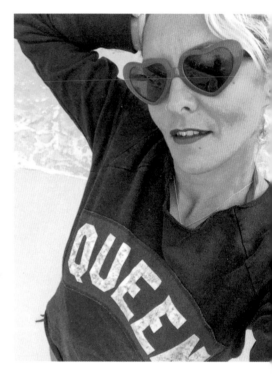

C ontrary to what you might think, being photogenic is not a gift. There are tips for taking good photos every time:

1 PLAY WITH **LIGHT**

Photography is about lighting, more than anything. Natural daylight—if you avoid direct sunlight—is always best, it's more flattering for your skin than artificial light. If you're inside, place yourself near a source of light. However be careful not to overexpose your face: this will erase details and the photo will be too light (it will look washed out). On the other hand, if your photo is too dark, or underexposed, we won't see you. Take a few test shots ahead of time.

Forget about taking selfies at night: there is not enough light and you'll have to use the flash, which will surely make you look like a vampire. If you absolutely must, use the soft, bluish glow of your computer screen as a source of light, which will produce an interesting effect on the face.

When preparing a professional photo shoot, the photographer often calls for a stand-in. This allows the team to test and adjust the lighting in keeping with the poses the model will be doing for the shoot once the technical tests have been done. It's a precious timesaver!

2 PAY ATTENTION TO THE **BACKGROUND**

The decor around you is important. A busy background can ruin a good photo. Choose a dark, clean background. In your home, it could be a door, for example. In the street, a wall of a harmonious color. Avoid standing in front of people who are moving around or places that are too full of movement. This can create a disorderly background that will be detrimental to the result you are seeking.

"PHOTOGRAPHY IS AN ATTITUDE, A WAY OF EXISTING, A WAY OF LIFE."

HENRI CARTIER-BRESSON

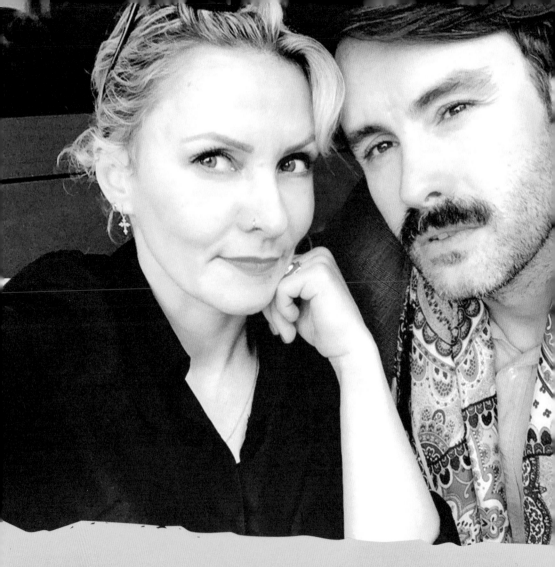

THE POINT OF THE **SELFIE** IS TO **HIGHLIGHT** YOUR **FACE**

- Wear lipstick or gloss.
- Use a little blush so you'll have a healthy glow.
- Use corrector to minimize the gray areas of your face.

- Pay attention to how you are dressed: go for the colors that will bring out your complexion and favor a neat over a sloppy look.

PROFESSIONAL ADVICE

Practice in front of a mirror to determine which angles make you prettiest, and repeat this in front of the lens. In the 1990s, the greatest top models asked that a mirror be placed behind the photographer so they could adjust their expressions.

How will you know if you've found your best? By the many compliments you'll receive when you show your photos!

4 **"SMILE**, YOU'RE ON CAMERA!"
Forget the sad face and the frown! There is nothing like a radiant smile or crooked little grin. Remember your old class photos, where the photographer asked you to say "cheese" to turn your sullen expression into a happy, lively smile.

Once again, less is more: don't exaggerate. Stay natural. If you force yourself, you'll look tense and your photo won't be good. There is nothing like spontaneity.

Also forget the pouty look, the famous "duck face" (you know the one I mean, the little puckered smirk that makes you look so smart) that abounds on social networks.

The key is in the eyes: for a photo to be good, you have to be happy in it. Don't be afraid to charm your camera: in selfie mode, it is your best friend. Look straight into the lens and be sure of yourself.

3 FIND JUST THE **RIGHT ANGLE**
Everything is a question of perspective: a photo taken from above will make you look slimmer but could deform you so you look like an extraterrestrial (big forehead, small chin), while a photo taken from below will give you the impression of having a double chin and will make your body look wider. And that's not what we're going for.

So the best position is to hold your smartphone or camera straight in front of you, slightly high, an arms' length away. Facing the camera, don't hesitate to do tests to find the position you like best, where you look the most beautiful. The ¾ angle is the one models use most for selfies, like for fashion and beauty shoots. Arm on hip, slightly away from your body. Try it. Above all, to keep it harmonious, don't zoom too much onto your face.

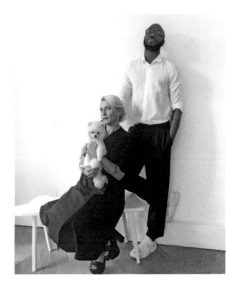

17

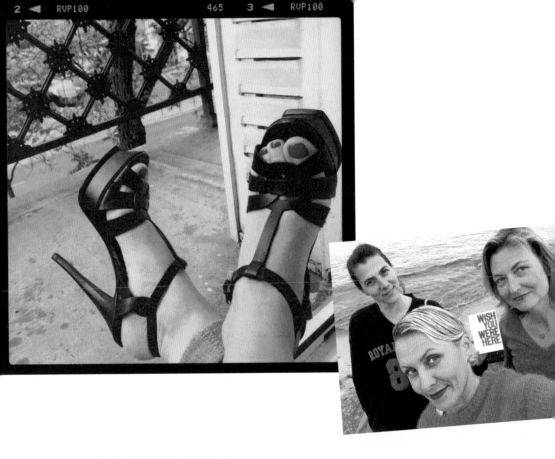

5 AIRBRUSH YOUR SELFIE

If the dark circles under your eyes are too pronounced, your complexion is too dull, or you have a blemish in the middle of your forehead, you can retouch your photo (it's recommended!). There are lots of apps to help you do this (Facetune, for example). Be careful, as with everything else, not to overdo it. If it's too airbrushed, you'll look disguised, like a doll.

6 USE FILTERS

Sepia, black and white, vintage–have fun trying filters on your selfie and finding the color that offers the best embellishment. All the photo apps now have many of them. Try them and use the one you like the best!

7 FINALLY, POST IT!

Don't be selfish: after you've taken such a pretty selfie, you have to share it!

IN GROUP SHOTS

You have to squeeze together to fit into the frame! This is when everyone has to put on their best face. In this case, the famous "selfie stick," which lengthens tourists' arms, is very useful.

POST YOUR FAVORITE SELFIE.
\# #getgorgeous, #beautychallenge21

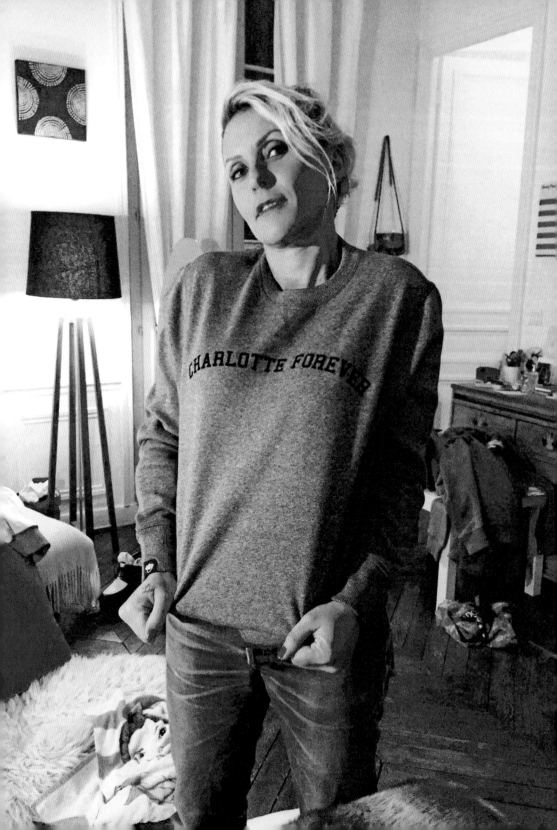

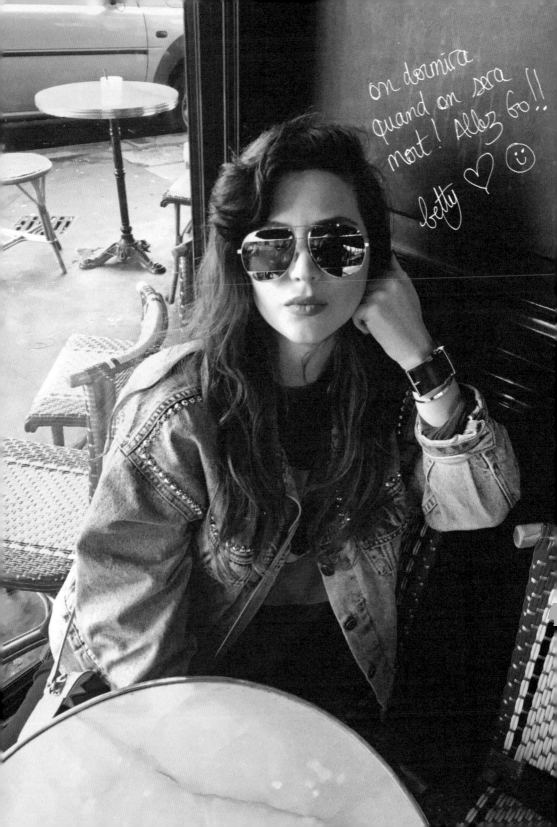

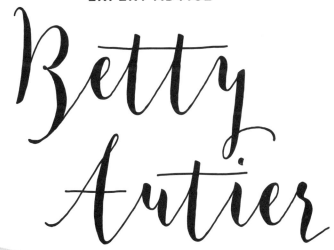

Betty Autier

AGE: 32

PROFESSION: Influencer/Instagrammer

YOUR FIRST JOB: Sales clerk at Etam

YOUR FAVORITE PHOTO OF YOURSELF: One of my first photos posted on the Internet, with my bangs falling over my eyes and a big smile

ASTROLOGICAL SIGN: Libra

DISTINGUISHING FEATURE: I was a vegetarian for twenty years and I switched sides in 2014

WHAT CAN'T YOU LIVE WITHOUT: My friends!

WHAT DO YOU DO AS A SPECIAL TREAT FOR YOURSELF? Go out to restaurants with my friends, then spend the rest of the night out having fun with them

YOUR THREE SIGNATURE WARDROBE PIECES: My vintage Thriller jacket, flat Giuseppe Zanotti glitter leather ankle boots, and Schott bomber jacket

THREE MUST-HAVE BEAUTY PRODUCTS: Estée Lauder foundation, Nars Orgasm blush, taupe eye shadow from M·A·C

YOUR PERFUME: I change perfumes all the time; my latest: Dior's Fahrenheit

WHO IS YOUR IDOL: Michael Jackson

WHAT BOOK IS ON YOUR NIGHTSTAND: Robert Cialdini's *Influence: The Psychology of Persuasion*

YOUR LUCKY CHARM: A Brazilian Senhor do Bonfim bracelet

LESS OR MORE: More!!

YOUR MOTTO: "Let's go!"

YOUR ADVICE FOR READERS: Try to do as little as possible to please others and learn to assert yourself as much as possible. People like following those who are sure of themselves!

How did you get the idea to do a blog? I was an actress in the Cours Florent drama school and I wanted to put the photos from my book on the Internet. I kind of just stumbled upon the blog format by accident!

Are you a selfie addict? I like to do selfies but I'm not what you'd call an addict. I try to be on good behavior in social situations!

Selfies: Ego trip or self-love? I would say it's a way of loving yourself and perfectly controlling your image. It's a little boost to the ego and we all need that.

The three golden rules for taking a good selfie:
1. Stand facing a source of natural light.
2. Raise the smartphone a little for an angle that slims the face.
3. Also pout a little, to make a duck face! It's key!

With Instagram and Snapchat now, everybody has started blogging. What has this changed for you? Because of Instagram and Snapchat, blogs have become old hat. I stopped doing mine and I find these new ways of communicating to be more of a reflex and much more fun.

What top photographer would you like to pose for? I fulfilled my dream when I posed for Terry Richardson! I am going to think of my next target.

———

Facing page: We'll sleep when we're dead. Let's go!!

DAY

18

BEING A SMART

Shopper

ELIMINATE FASHION DON'TS

DESIGNERS
AS SOURCES
OF **INSPIRATION**

"Whoever said money can't buy happiness
simply didn't know where to go shopping."

Bo Derek

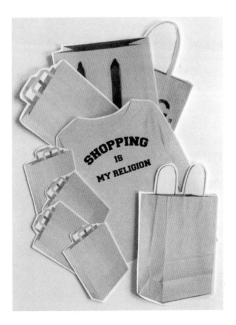

S hopping is the activity of the century!
Who hasn't dreamed of going on a
shopping spree, like Julia Roberts did
in *Pretty Woman?* Of course we associate
shopping with spending money, but, above
all, it's a woman's sport, an unending source
of good times shared between mother and
daughter or among friends. Far more than
providing a solution to the need for clothes,
shopping sets the stage for dreaming. That's
why we can go into a gorgeous shop to try
on a dress we don't always have the money
for, simply for the pleasure of trying it on.

Nothing can compare to the times I go
along with top models to choose what they
will wear for a soirée or a red-carpet event. I
have great memories of these times, like when
Azzedine Alaïa himself came to greet us when
we were trying something on in his studio.

Shopping isn't necessarily a question of
money, and today you can shop online—I
am thinking particularly of all the private
sales websites that exist, clearance sales, the
closet clear-out sales—and you can find
bargains all year. Yet with so many options
to choose from, how can you keep your head
from spinning?

18

THE **GOLDEN RULES**
OF SMART SHOPPING

1 KNOW WHAT LOOKS **GOOD ON YOU**

This is rule number 1. The secret to smart shopping lies in good self-awareness. As we have already said (*see* Day 1), it's important to look at yourself honestly, to quietly consider your good features and your flaws. The idea, above all, is not to fight yourself and your body type, but on the contrary to highlight your good features and hide your flaws. Several times throughout this book, I've mentioned that not even the world's best models have a perfect body. So be realistic and don't lie to yourself. There is no point in convincing yourself that size 6 looks good on you if you're a size 10! What's important is not to look thin, but to feel beautiful and elegant, and buying clothes that are not the right size is a waste of time and money. Knowing yourself well is also being aware of the shapes and colors that suit you. Make the effort to remember the compliments you received when wearing certain clothes. These compliments are often more trustworthy than your reflection in the mirror. This is why it is often useful when you are shopping to bring a friend with you (a real friend) who will know how to help you make good choices.

2 DON'T ALLOW YOURSELF TO **BE INFLUENCED**

Though it's not always the case, sometimes you have to be wary of what salespeople tell you, as they can say anything to prompt you to make a purchase, and you'll forget what's essential:
- Do you need this piece of clothing?
- Does it really look that great on you?

This is why I strongly encourage you to go shopping with a friend and, above all, give yourself time to think. Tell yourself that the pants that you did not at all plan on buying will not go away from one day to the next; keep the pants in mind and if, in a few days, you still want them, you can go back to the store or buy them online. Rest assured that not all of my purchases are planned, and sometimes I, too, give in. I remember caving in last season when I saw a pair of wedges in the Jimmy Choo shop window. I told myself it wasn't very reasonable, but I stepped into the shop anyway. Twenty minutes later, under the spell of a warm welcome, a cheerful atmosphere, lively music, and a free glass of champagne, I left with two pairs of shoes!

But don't forget: you and you alone are the one who decides!

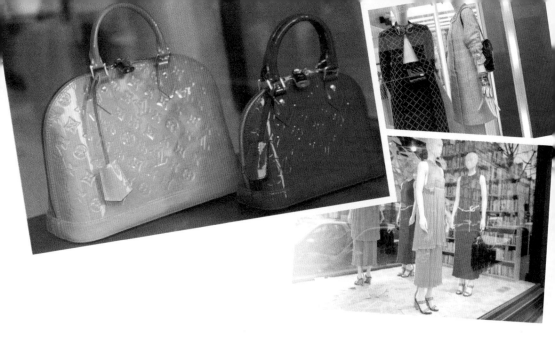

3 THINK BEFORE YOU BUY

Impulse buying is fun, it's good for the morale and it gives you a high. Yet remember that a wardrobe is something you build up (*see* Day 5). Like a collector, you are going to search out the pieces you lack, and you're going to seek out those worn-out items you liked very much. So it's long-term work that requires a bit of patience. I recommend you check the websites of the brands you're interested in. It's a great timesaver. Online multibrand stores like Net-à-Porter and Asos are also very interesting, and you'll find they carry new labels. The fashion press is full of excellent shopping advice that will help you make choices before heading into action. Beyond seasons and trends, think about choosing pieces that go together over the long term, enabling you gradually to build your style, your identity.

4 BE WARY OF BARGAINS

We are all bombarded by daily notifications about special promotional items, good deals, and private sales, not to mention the seasonal sales. Buying at inexpensive prices is good, but be careful not to buy just anything, under the pretext that it was a good deal. Like me, you have probably already bought clothes in the sales in a color not exactly suited to your taste or in the wrong size. Why? When you think about it, there's absolutely no point to this. Price is a key element in decision-making, but it must not guide everything. It is better to wait a little, even at high prices, and buy that handbag you've been dreaming of, the one you'll keep several years, rather than to jump on a cheaper model that you don't really want.

18

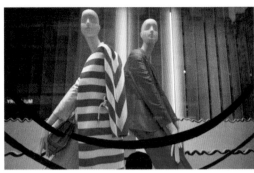

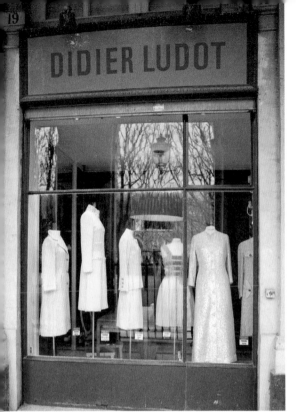

6 MIX **CHEAP** WITH **CHIC**

What should we think about "fast fashion"? Let's be honest. What we would do without Zara and H&M? I only know a handful of women, including those in the fashion world, who refuse to buy clothes from these chain stores. Obviously, the economic model is clearly based on the copy—sometimes literally—of "real" designer collections, and this is rather upsetting, ethically. While you can't deny that the style/price ratio they offer defies competition, I still don't encourage you to build your wardrobe at these magnates of fast fashion. For one thing, their clothes are not known for durability, and for another, it's difficult to mask, for a total look, where the clothes come from.

As you can well imagine, subtlety lies in the art of mixing and matching, which is also the best way of creating doubt and to make it seem that an inexpensive piece is a designer item. Buy quality-brand basics and add inexpensive seasonal pieces to them from time to time.

Now you can make some real purchases that you have thought about and that are useful, without spending a fortune. These common-sense rules don't keep you from caving in to temptation from time to time, either, and from treating yourself to something special, because after all that's what shopping is all about.

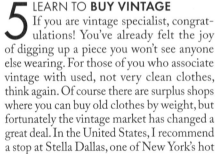

5 LEARN TO **BUY VINTAGE**

If you are vintage specialist, congratulations! You've already felt the joy of digging up a piece you won't see anyone else wearing. For those of you who associate vintage with used, not very clean clothes, think again. Of course there are surplus shops where you can buy old clothes by weight, but fortunately the vintage market has changed a great deal. In the United States, I recommend a stop at Stella Dallas, one of New York's hot vintage boutiques (285 N 6th St, Brooklyn, N.Y. 11211). In fact, more and more stores offer clothes in good shape, organized by category and by color, while many prestigious brands—Ralph Lauren, Urban Outfitters, and APC (with its famous jeans)—are developing lines of freshened up vintage clothes. Don't hesitate to check them out!

POST YOUR BEST SHOPPING FIND.

\# #getgorgeous, #beautychallenge21

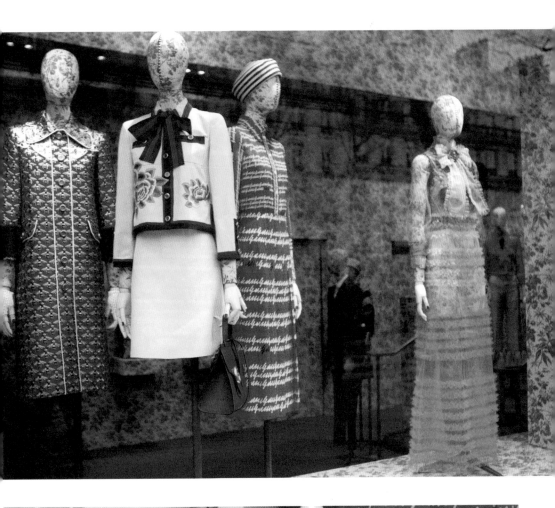
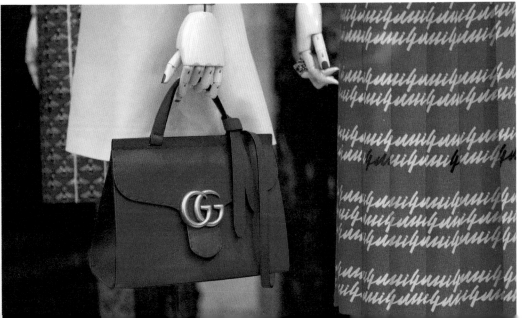

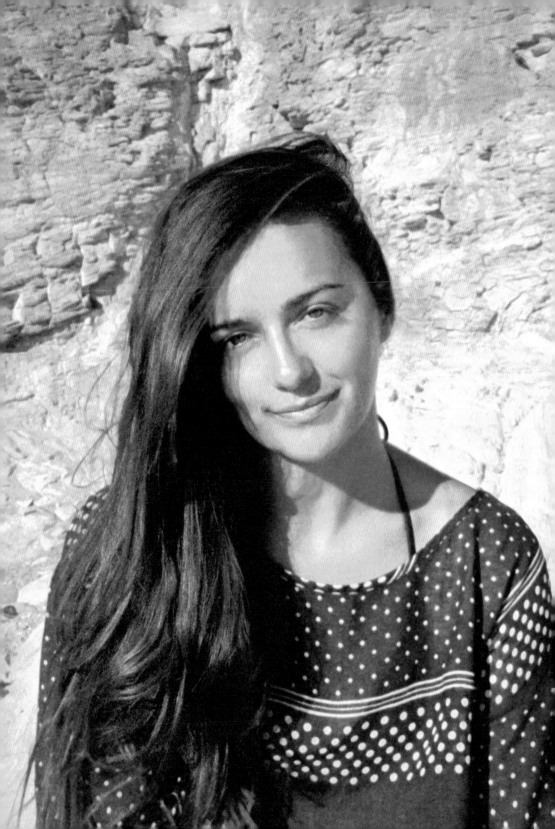

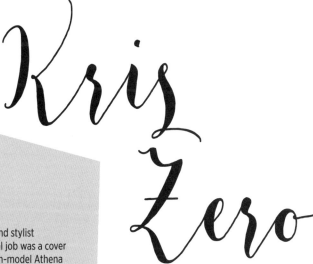

Kris Zero

AGE: 33
PROFESSION: Fashion editor and stylist
FIRST JOB: My first big editorial job was a cover for *Anthem Magazine* with then-model Athena Currey; after that came *Teen Vogue*, *10*, and *Muse*
YOUR FAVORITE PHOTO OF YOURSELF: Any picture where I'm on the beach; it's my happy place
ASTROLOGICAL SIGN: Virgo
DISTINGUISHING FEATURE: Big brows
WHAT CAN'T YOU LIVE WITHOUT: Road trips
WHAT DO YOU DO AS A SPECIAL TREAT FOR YOURSELF? Surf, cook, or—when I have more than a day—take a road trip. I like getting outside into nature or spending time at home with friends.
YOUR THREE SIGNATURE WARDROBE PIECES: Proenza Schouler poncho, The Elder Statesman sweater, anything by Ulla Johnson
THREE MUST-HAVE BEAUTY PRODUCTS: I go super natural: my favorite skin care *anything* comes from Living Libations, I love the lip tint from Fat and the Moon, and, if I wear makeup at all, it's from RMS Beauty
YOUR PERFUME: I use essential oils; I love sandalwood
WHO IS YOUR IDOL: Kids, they know best how to live in the moment
WHAT BOOK IS ON YOUR NIGHTSTAND: My dream journal
YOUR LUCKY CHARM: A shell ring that I've worn for years
LESS OR MORE: Way less
YOUR MOTTO: "Live in the moment."
YOUR ADVICE FOR READERS: Be yourself, and your style will always be more dynamic and interesting than if you try to be someone else.

Designers or fast fashion? I don't think it's one or the other; it's about affordability. And don't forget vintage!
Are you a compulsive or calculated shopper? Never compulsive. Never too calculated. I like spontaneous shopping. You see something in a window, and you know you're going to feel good when you have it on!
What is the biggest shopping "don't": Don't overdo it on trends.
Your favorite shopping city: Tokyo; you can find the craziest, most unique stuff!
Advice for how to be a smart shopper: Spend your time and energy looking for what you *need*. We all have too many of one thing and not enough of something else!
Why is shopping important? More importantly, I think the question should be "why is fashion important"? It's expression! A first impression! And for many of us, it's a personal, daily art.

01
02
03
04
05
06
07
08
09
10
11
12
13
14
15
16
17
18
19
20
21

DAY

19

IMPROVING MY

Lifestyle

TAKE CARE OF THE DETAILS IN MY SURROUNDINGS

MY HOME REFLECTS WHO I AM

"Existing is a fact, living is an art."

Frédéric Lenoir

The art of living is a vast, personal idea. I wouldn't presume to make recommendations about how you should live, but I will try to give you the keys to finding your ideal lifestyle, the one you feel is just right for you.

Let's switch the words around to come up with a definition of the art of living: "to live for art." I like this idea: seeking elegance, beauty, harmony, and quality around you and putting quantity in the back seat. Believe me, it does a world of good.

When you think about it, the efforts you make to look gorgeous and have style—unless you spend your life in front of a mirror—benefit the people around you more than yourself. That's why it's important to think a little about ourselves by ensuring that our daily surroundings, in particular our home interior, is the extension of the image we have been cultivating since we took up this challenge.

As we have already mentioned (*see* Day 5), it is essential for you to stake a claim to your home interior, to fashion it, as you see fit, to create a welcoming, comforting, and visually pleasing setting. We spend lots of time in our home. So it's useless to add to the daily stresses of life with an interior that is a badly lit, non-functional, anxiety-provoking mess.

It's been a long time since I've thought of housework as a chore. Every weekend, just like for my body, my hair, and my skin, I make an appointment with myself for a kind of ritual in which my house becomes mine again. I reconcile myself to the place that, during the week, with the help of my children and cats, turned into a kind of lion's den where everything piled up and the kitchen cabinets emptied out as fast as the laundry basket filled up.

SO HERE ARE
A **FEW TIPS**

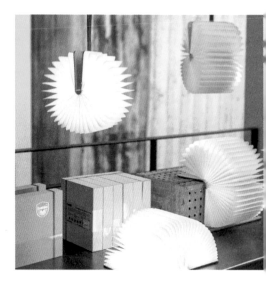

1 CREATE **SPACE**
This is one of the fundamental rules when it comes to decoration. We all lead very busy daily lives. So let's give our brain the calm space it needs, starting by giving it a visual rest. Without obsessing over it, I like my house to be in order and for everything to be in place—it keeps crisis moments at bay, believe me.

Collecting is a great decoration idea when it is intentional and clearly thought out. However, collecting things to collect them serves no purpose; it creates confusion and fills up the little bit of room you have when you live in a small space. Sometimes you have to know how to create an empty space.

If you have a touch of the hoarder in you, invest in pretty boxes to hide everything that doesn't deserve to be seen.

2 SHINE A LITTLE **LIGHT**
Whether on the catwalk, at the theater, or in the movies, lighting is one of the major features of stage design. With it we can highlight certain key points, warm up the setting, or, on the contrary, cool it down. There is no point spending lots of money on decoration if the lighting is not carefully thought out.

As with photos (*see* Day 17), natural lighting creates the best effect, but there are lots of solutions if it's lacking. It's always better to double up on secondary light sources than to have a central source that's too harsh. Several low-intensity lamps will give your living room or bedroom a cozy feel.

Don't forget, however, that some rooms, like the kitchen or, of course, the bathroom require more intense lighting. If you don't want to get depressed when you look in the mirror, use a white, diffuse light source (not spotlights, which will make your complexion look awful and will be of no help when applying makeup).

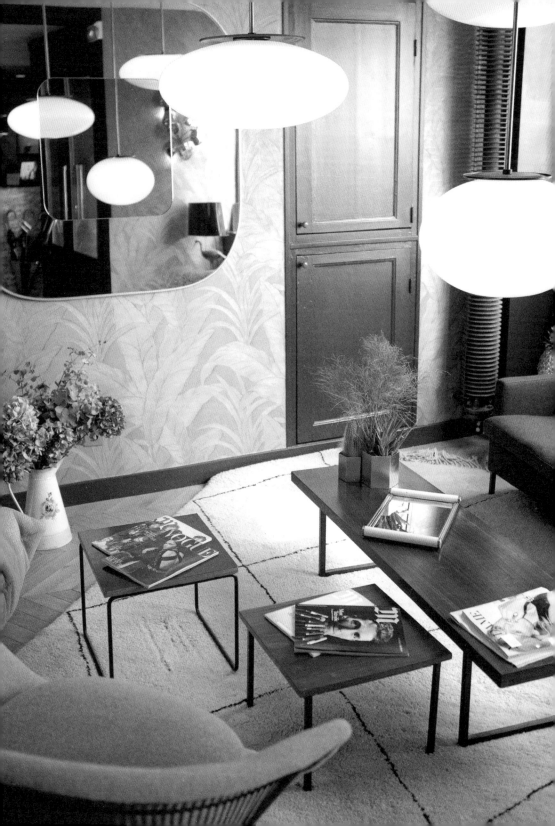

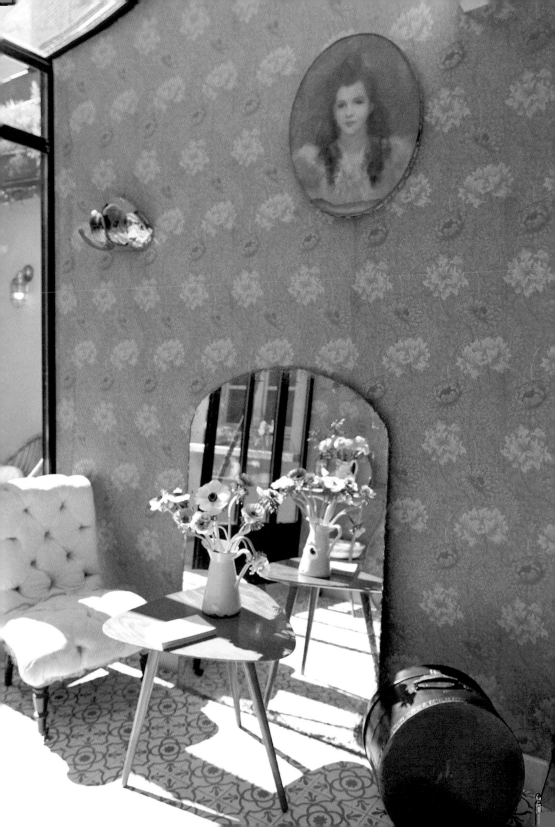

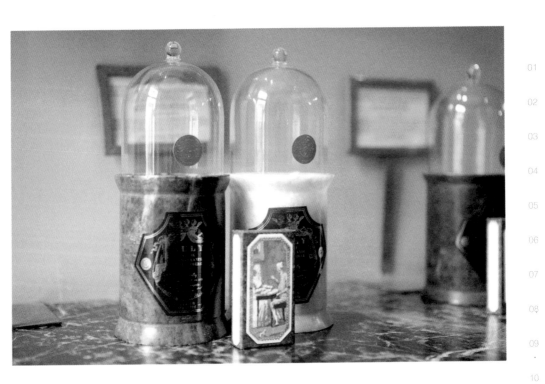

3 FRESHEN THINGS UP WITH ROOM **FRAGRANCE**

As we have previously stated, a subtly scented home is an invitation to serenity (*see* Day 11). What advice is there for creating your signature home fragrance? Scented candles like those from Diptyque, Cire Trudon, and Buly L'Officine Universelle are fabulous. You can also burn incense sticks or incense papers like Santa Maria Novella's, or add a few drops of essential oil to your dust rag. Don't forget it's very pleasant to scent your bath, bed linens, and closet with essential oils. For a more pronounced fragrance signature, you can use sparing amounts of home scents like Nicolaï's.

4 GO **BARGAIN-HUNTING**

I'm not a fan of the word "personalization," which we hear on every home-decoration show, but I find the idea interesting. There's no point having a perfectly decorated interior if the soul and spirit of the people who live in the place are not apparent. So to avoid the impersonal, "too perfect" look or simply to give a little life to your IKEA furniture, go out in search of things that make your home unique, like you. Like for clothes and accessories (*see* Day 18), nosing around to uncover that rare find is really worth it, and it's money well spent. So head to the flea market and antiques stores and zoom around on eBay.com, a real gold mine.

19

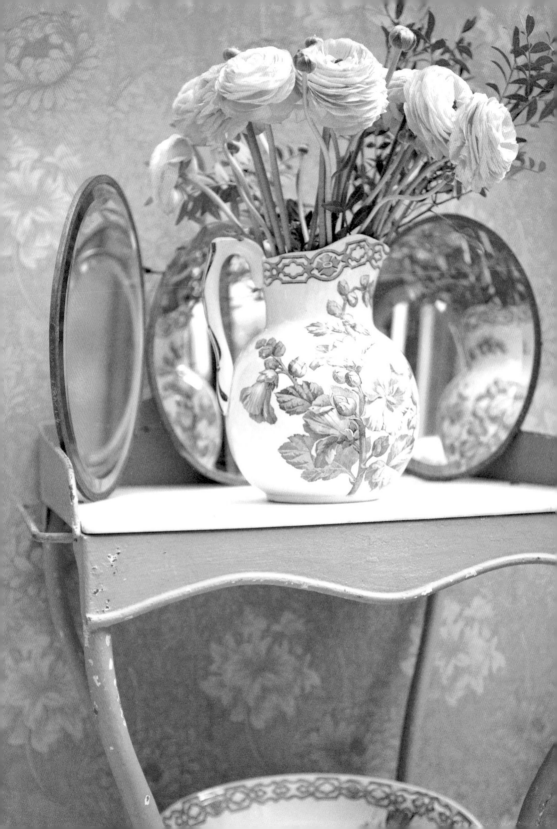

CHRISTEL'S LITTLE RITUAL

When I wake up, or before I turn in for the night, I make myself turn off all screens (telephone, TV, computer, etc.) and listen to classical music: the soothing effect is guaranteed.

7 SET THE **STAGE**

Your interior is the closed-door theater of your personal life. Don't hesitate to pretend you're a stage director to make your space more welcoming and friendly. Create special areas and nooks for each member of your family. We all need our own special territory. So it's important, when you live with others, to create private spaces, whether an office space, a bathroom, a closet, or a boudoir (*see* Day 5). It is also of primary importance to think about the communal spaces, where people talk and share things; it's nice for everyone to be able to sit at the same table or relax together in the living room. To do that, think of extra chairs and big cushions, so that the whole family can feel at ease.

5 BUY **FLOWERS**

Plants are good, provided you have a green thumb. They can also be a bit monotonous—there's all that greenery that settles into your decor. For me, there's nothing like the bucolic charm of a bouquet of flowers, whether a gift or a treat for yourself. Offering yourself to a pretty seasonal bouquet every week or simply picking a few flowers when you're out on a stroll in the country is an excellent way to please yourself and introduce a bit of serenity at home. Aside from being pretty to look at, they give your interior a lively, romantic note: don't hold back!

6 LISTEN TO **MUSIC**

Lighting may help create atmosphere and make a house look lively, but you can't neglect music, either. Silence is sometimes golden, but it can also be sad and anxiety-provoking. Music has recognized soothing effects. It can be cheerful or melancholic, soft or energetic: it's easy to find music to suit your mood.

Create playlists on Soundcloud or Deezer, for example, and listen to them in relaxing moments at home. If you are into vintage, invest in a record player and vinyl records, which will give a very trendy retro touch to your decor.

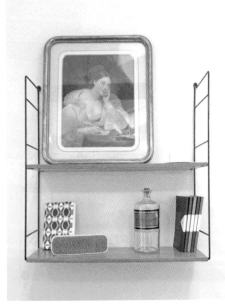

19

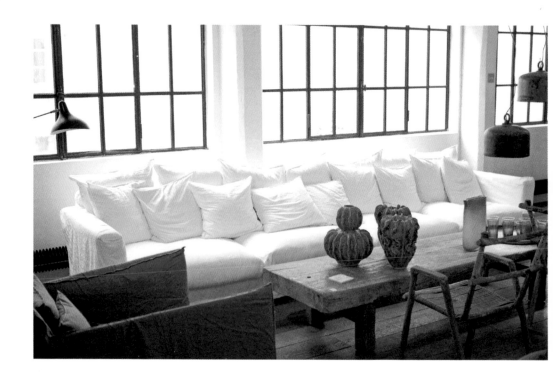

8 RECEIVE **GUESTS**

Whether your apartment is large enough to hold a big dinner or more suited to pre-dinner drinks and hors d'oeuvres with a small group of friends, remember your home must always be pleasant for your visitors. You can bargain-hunt for mismatched antique tableware and silver by weight (not expensive at flea markets), light candles, open a good bottle of wine (the one your friends like). If you decide to serve up a last-minute dinner, there are restaurants and apps that offer home deliveries of your favorite meals. Pamper your guests, double up on little details and special treatment. That's what the art of living is all about. What good does it do to have impeccable style if you don't behave with elegance and generosity toward others? Plus, offering a nice moment to friends in the privacy of your home is another way of being good to yourself, as well.

9 **GO OUT**

If, after all this advice you don't feel like leaving your home, it means I've won the bet. Yet in spite of it all, the art of living is also knowing how to choose the right places to go for lunch with friends, for a romantic dinner, or to drink a few cocktails. A piece of advice: take control of the situation, don't let anyone take you to a place you don't like. To spend good times with your friends, choosing the right place counts a lot. Pick out the little restaurant with beautiful lighting for dinner, the pretty sunny terrace for lunch, or the bar with elegant customers for a drink. There's no use dressing to the nines only to find you're in a place where everyone is dressed down. That would be bizarre. To avoid that, seek out the best addresses and create habits going to places you like. In short, be an aesthete!

POST YOUR FAVORITE INTERIOR SHOT.

#getgorgeous, #beautychallenge21

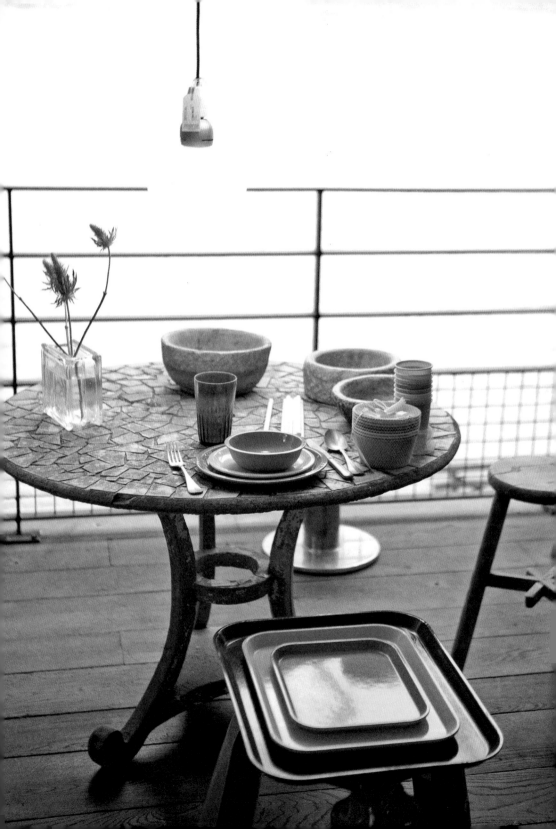

Why not !

Margherita Missoni

AGE: 33
PROFESSION: Owner and designer at Margherita Kids
FIRST JOB: *Vogue Paris* intern, at 15 years old
YOUR FAVORITE PHOTO OF YOURSELF: A portrait
taken twenty years ago by Gilles Bensimon
ASTROLOGICAL SIGN: Pisces
DISTINGUISHING FEATURE: Naturally great eyebrows
WHAT CAN'T YOU LIVE WITHOUT: Ice cream
WHAT DO YOU DO AS A SPECIAL TREAT FOR
YOURSELF: Take a hot bath with 4 ½ lbs. (2 kg) of salt
YOUR THREE SIGNATURE WARDROBE
PIECES: YSL trench coat, Missoni space-dyed
cashmere sweater, Levi's® 501 jeans
THREE MUST-HAVE BEAUTY PRODUCTS: Lucas'
Papaw ointment, Nuxe Huile Prodigieuse®
Or Shimmering Dry Oil, cream blush
YOUR PERFUME: Songes by Annick Goutal
WHO IS YOUR IDOL: Tina Modotti, the Italian
actress, model, photographer, and activist
WHAT BOOK IS ON YOUR NIGHTSTAND:
Just Kids by Patti Smith
YOUR LUCKY CHARM: A glass pendant
containing hair from my babies; it was a
present from my dear Zac Posen
LESS OR MORE: Lately, less
YOUR MOTTO: "Why not?!"
WHAT ADVICE WOULD YOU GIVE
READERS: Give it a chance.

Is your style an extension of your lifestyle? Yes.
**How do you describe the way you live
your life?** I put serenity first.
**Do you pay as much attention to how your living
space looks as you do to your own look?** Yes.
**Is your home pristine, like something out of a
magazine, or is it more "lived in"?** Lived in.
**What advice would you give for creating a cozy
atmosphere at home?** Build it around your habits.
What is your current home decor fetish? Wallpapers.

DAY

20

STAYING

Current

TRENDSPOTTING

CULTIVATE YOUR **MIND!**

"**Magazine:** Eighteenth century.
Borrowed from the French word magasin.
Illustrated periodical publication, generally weekly,
dealing with various subjects."

Dictionnaire de l'Académie Française

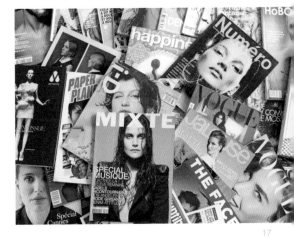

I mproving your knowledge and being curious means you stay beautiful, because what is a body without life inside? Having a lively mind, thinking, reading, writing, and endeavoring to have a good soul are all beauty recommendations. Having gorgeous skin and beautiful clothes are not enough for excelling in high society. I remember one of the books I read that made the biggest impression on me when I was very young and still shaping my personality: *The Picture of Dorian Gray* by Oscar Wilde. This fascinating tale was a revelation to me: that it is impossible to separate the soul from the envelope of the body.

Eileen Ford, founder of one of the world's first modeling agencies, gave precious advice to the models she recruited, putting up some of them in her own home, to give them a bit of polish. Rigor, discipline, and reading were part of the program set up by the person that supermodels Naomi Campbell, Christy Turlington, and others can thank.

The print media is still one of the ways of becoming informed. Today, even though information is everywhere and culture available to everyone via the Internet, paper has resisted and shouldn't be neglected in favor of online navigation. Actually it seems that the competition has been beneficial and that, as a catalyst, the Internet has revolutionized the print media and is spurring it to evolve and keep improving its quality.

20

WHAT **MAGAZINES** SHOULD I **BUY**?

Around age thirteen, I started buying fashion magazines: *Elle,* of course, *Glamour,* and the French *20 Ans,* along with *The Face* and *i-D.* I found limitless inspiration in them.

I admit, today there so much on offer, so many fashion magazines, that it's difficult to choose. Let's proceed in stages.

WEEKLY STYLE SUPPLEMENTS

Like celebrity magazines such as *People* or *Us Weekly,* the French edition of *Elle* is published weekly. It has a more realistic approach to fashion and where you can sniff out great shopping ideas by mixing expensive and inexpensive items. A few years ago, *Elle* magazine appeared on Monday, and I wouldn't have missed it for anything! It was a way of starting the week with a club of "girlfriends," those journalists who gave me such precious advice.

Similarly, Sunday styles sections, such as *The New York Times's T Magazine* or *The Telegraph's Stella* magazine, help create a tight bond with the public; readers look forward to receiving their weekly issues. I have great affection for these weeklies and, whatever happens, *Elle* will always be *Elle,* a real institution. But the Internet offers serious competition, because apart from the special fashion editions, these magazines are not meant to be kept. So it's tempting to read them online, it costs less, and it's more eco-friendly.

MONTHLIES

I wouldn't be able to start this paragraph without talking about *Vogue.* As soon as it was launched in 1909 in New York, the magazine, which was bimonthly at the time, became *the* fashion bible. It was a religion in its own right, with its grand, famous priestesses: Diana Vreeland and Anna Wintour for the American edition, Edmonde Charles-Roux and Carine Roitfeld for the French one, and Anna Piaggi and Franca Sozzani for the Italian.

Vogue is very frankly oriented to luxury—the real deal—often out of reach for ordinary mortals. Being able to afford them is of little importance, because the magazine allows us to dream. In the end, when you think about it, it's a wonderful idea: skimming through the magazine guarantees an escape from your daily life in a few seconds. Like a novel that takes you on an adventure, *Vogue* offers a journey into what fashion does best, a kind of fairytale told by the greatest stylists, models, and photographers. An inexhaustible source of inspiration, I've collected this magazine since the age of eighteen and it has never stopped feeding my creativity.

There's a detail of the *Vogue* layout that I really like: every edition has a white spine bearing the famous black logo, an invitation to collect them. They look great displayed on a shelf in the living room—I know I never tire of them!

"*VOGUE* IS A FASHION MAGAZINE, AND A FASHION MAGAZINE IS ABOUT CHANGE."

ANNA WINTOUR

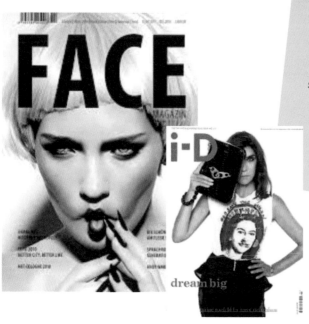

If *Vogue* and its overt luxury bent don't do it for you, try hipper monthlies. Check out the two iconic British magazines *i-D Magazine* and *Dazed & Confused*, and the legendary American magazines *Interview*, founded by Andy Warhol in 1969, and *W Magazine* as well.

MOOKS

This term is a portmanteau of "magazine" and "book." It's a periodicals category that has really taken off in the past few years, in total opposition to Internet offers. Issued quarterly, biannually, or yearly, mooks are much more "in your face" with their look borrowed from art books. Large format, they are bound like real books, printed on beautiful paper and feature a card stock cover. They may be expensive, but they are designed to be collected and are an integral part of your decor (*see* Day 19). You will always be pleased, even after ten years, to skim through these big, image-filled mooks. Purists will go as far as buying the same issue, published with different covers.

There are many mooks available today, and new titles are created every year. Among my favorites is the French magazine *Égoïste*, started in 1977 by Nicole Wisniak, with its very large format and custom-made ads, whose vintage editions are now worth their weight in gold. I love *Self Service* and Ezra Petronio's famous *Polaroids*, and the beautiful magazine *Antidote* edited by my friend Yann Weber. I am so proud to have supported him by offering him my best models when he was launching it a few years ago. Another favorite is Katie Grand's very pop *Love Magazine* with a super fresh perspective, offering a fun, nutty view of fashion that does a lot of good. Of course, there's the unforgettable and very inspiring *CR Fashion Book* by Madame Carine Roitfeld herself!

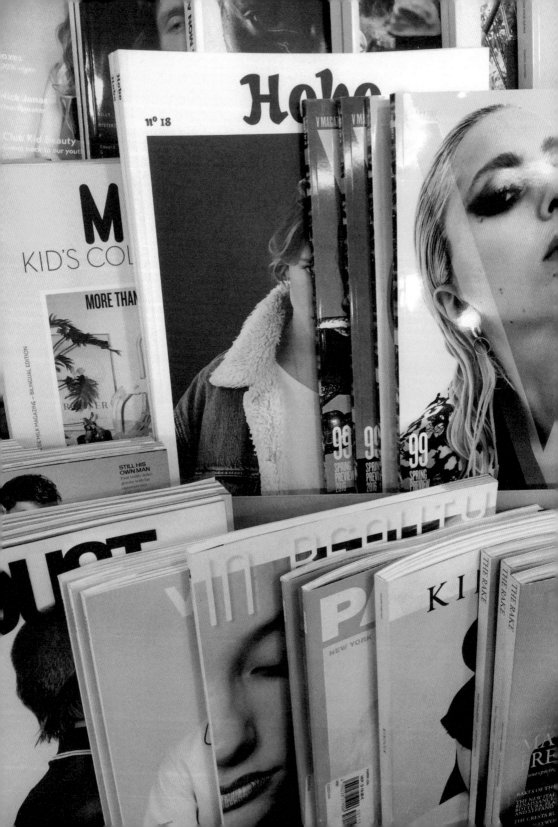

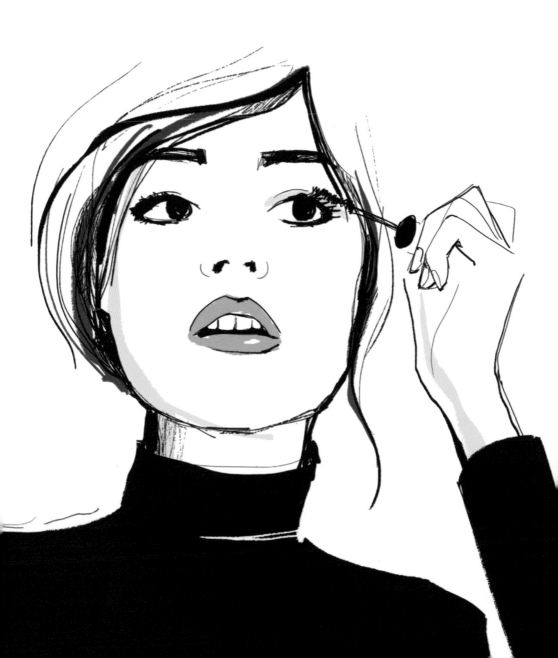

HOW TO FIND
MY WAY AROUND
ONLINE

E ven if, like me, you're not part of the digital generation or a "digital native"—born into the Internet age—you know, of course, that using the Internet is now essential. Sorting through online choices is key.

ONLINE MAGAZINES
Internet versions of paper magazines are interesting because their content is constantly updated. All fashion magazines now have a Smartphone app, so—to keep informed in public transportation systems, for example—you can download the pages that interest you in advance and check them whenever you want, even without a network connection!

• models.com: The bible of modeling agencies. A kind of directory in which you can find models by category, and where you can also find the latest fashion campaigns.

• vogue.com: The American *Vogue* website is a real treasure trove, featuring images from all of the fashion shows, season by season.

• nowfashion.com: For watching fashion shows live, as if you were there in person.

• fashioncopious.com: If you don't want to miss any fashion series or the latest ad campaigns.

BLOGS
They were the subject of debate when they were just emerging a few years ago, and professional journalists were sometimes afraid that they would lose business to bloggers. Today the playing field has leveled. We have all become bloggers thanks to social media. In spite of all this, however, some blogs continue to capture readers' attention—garancedore.fr, thesartorialist.com, the French blog leblogdebetty.com, and rookiemag.com by the very hip Tavi Gevinson are favorites.

20

DESIGN
MY OWN **MAGAZINE**

As I just mentioned, social media has turned us all into bloggers. We post our photos and humorous messages daily. We create our own personal magazines, a window of expression.

Have fun carefully selecting the images you share, because your own blog is a real calling card. It has become a reflex to check the profiles of people you have just met or have an appointment to meet. Think about it.

SEVERAL **TOOLS**
ARE AT YOUR **FINGERTIPS**

• **TUMBLR**: Highly prized by creative types, who post texts, images, videos, links, and sound. The motto: "Post anything (from anywhere), customize everything, and find and follow what you love. Create your own Tumblr blog today."

• **PINTEREST**: More "girly" than Tumblr, it acts as an online mood board. It's easy to use and allows users to post and share ideas on their various centers of interest, passions, and hobbies through photo albums they've spotted online. The name of the site is a portmanteau of the words pin and interest. People love the photo album layout.

• **INSTAGRAM**: This app, which went live in 2010, has really boomed lately. Celebrities and major brands love it for being able to communicate quickly with images. By subscribing to the accounts of people who post content, you become a follower. Instagram has become a real barometer of popularity in the fashion world, and it's also an excellent way to expand your network of acquaintances.

• **SNAPCHAT**: The fashion world seized onto this app intended originally for teenagers, but that adults are totally crazy about. The very top magazines like *W* have created a Snapchat account. Their mini-videos bring us a step closer inside the private world of fashion people.

beautychallenge21
@Duo1321

422
Épingles

2K
J'aime

4K
Abonné

442
Abonnements

Day1
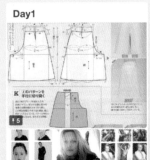
Modifier

Day2
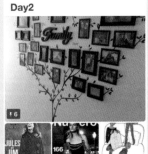
Modifier

Day3
COMMENT CREER UNE
MOODBOARD
*pour définir l' identité visuelle de
votre entreprise ou de votre blog*
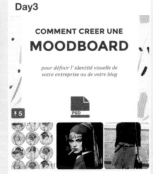
Modifier

Day4

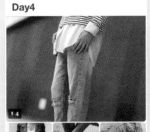
Modifier

Day5
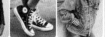
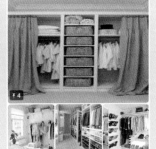
Modifier

Day6
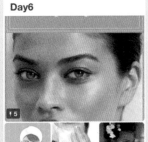
Modifier

Day7
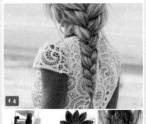
Modifier

Day8
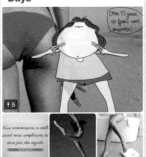
Modifier

Day9
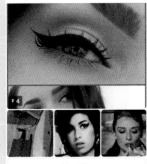
Modifier

TOO MUCH FASHION KILLS FASHION!

Even the most fashion crazed among us need to take a break from it. The top creative people will all tell you that you can't evolve in a vacuum, and that sources of inspiration must be constantly revived and can come from many different places. So to add to your world of fashion and style, get inspiration from outside the fashion world.

LISTEN TO MUSIC
Try websites like Deezer or Spotify, where you can listen to music files instantly; or on SoundCloud, a music-sharing platform I'm crazy about.

LOOK AROUND ONLINE
With the Internet, there are no more excuses not to improve your knowledge. To paraphrase Ferdinand Foch, Maréchal de France and member of the Académie Française: "There are no well-educated women, only women who educate themselves." Knowledge and the acquisition of knowledge are the work of a lifetime.

GO TO THE MOVIES
To dream and have a good time outside of your home. Movies: *c'est la vie!*

GO TO MUSEUMS
To take an imaginary journey, stimulate your senses, stir up unknown emotions. Art reveals beauty, and transforms those who allow themselves to get caught up in it. Without any useful purpose, art is a luxury that human beings cannot do without.

READ
To relax, to stimulate your brain, to escape. Whether novels, biographies, or classic works, take the time to hang out in bookstores and libraries to pick out some books.

GO TO THE THEATER OR THE OPERA
To experience emotions directly and for entertainment. Screens have invaded our space now. What a joy it is to have a good time, in person.

TAKE NOTES
Because writing is remembering. It is putting ideas and thoughts into words. Whether secrets in an intimate journal or simple notes in a weekly planner, take the time to write down whatever comes into your head.

DAY
20

Draft your "culture wishlist"

....
....
....
....
....
....
....
....
....
....
....
....
....
....

WHAT DID YOU DISCOVER TODAY?
\# #getgorgeous, #beautychallenge21

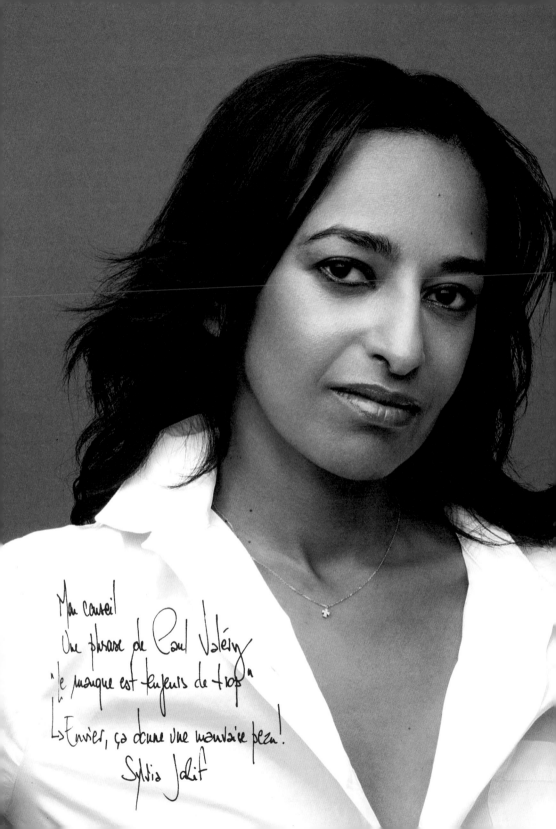

Mon conseil
Une phrase de Paul Valéry
"Le masque est toujours de trop"
↳ Envier, ça donne une mauvaise peau !
Sylvia Jolif

Sylvia Jorif

AGE: 46
PROFESSION: Head of fashion info
and journalist at *Elle* magazine
YOUR FIRST JOB: Reader for Éditions
François Bourin, when I was a student
YOUR FAVORITE PHOTOS OF YOURSELF:
Childhood photos from Trouville-sur-Mer,
where we vacationed every summer
ASTROLOGICAL SIGN: Gemini
YOU CAN'T LIVE WITHOUT: My contact
lenses because I'm very nearsighted
WHAT DO YOU DO AS A SPECIAL TREAT FOR
YOURSELF? Have a drink with my friends,
discover the city with my son, walk along the
seashore and watch the waves roll in and out
YOUR THREE SIGNATURE WARDROBE PIECES:
A little black dress, generally vintage, a navy
blue overcoat or pea coat, a shoulder bag
THREE MUST-HAVE BEAUTY PRODUCTS: Eucerin's
Ultra Sensitive Soin Apaisant Peau Sèche
day cream, Rino de Nicolo's Absolu Brillance
reconstructing hair mask with keratin, a tube of
Homéoplasmine®, the best balm for lips and any
little skin irritations (it's always in my bag)
YOUR PERFUME: I wear several, depending on
the season. In summer: L'Artisan Parfumeur's
Premier Figuier or Prada's Infusion de
Fleur d'Oranger. In winter: Balenciaga's
Paris or Chanel No. 5 Eau Première.
WHO IS YOUR IDOL: Marilyn Monroe
WHAT BOOK IS ON YOUR NIGHTSTAND: It's
impossible to choose only one! Raymond Queneau's
The Blue Flowers, Vladimir Nabokov's *Transparent
Things*, Marcel Proust's *Swann's Way*, and all my father
Richard Jorif's books, especially *Les Persistants Lilas*.
YOUR LUCKY CHARM: A photo booth shot of my son
at age four. The picture is always in my wallet. And a
small Virgin Mary that belonged to my grandmother.
LESS OR MORE: Less is more
YOUR MOTTO: "You don't need much to be happy."

Print or digital magazines? Print magazines,
absolutely. A print magazine is an object: you hold it
in your hand, take it with you on a trip, set it down,
pick it back up, skim through.... It establishes its own
timeframe, invites you to take a break, to concentrate.
**The first fashion magazine you ever
bought?** *Elle*, when I was a teenager,
discovering the top models of the 1980s.
Do you keep or toss magazines after reading? Both.
I have a big collection of *Elle* issues. In general I keep
the first issues of magazines, because they are full
of enthusiasm, starting energy, and a great spirit.
Your favorite magazines? Depending on the week,
Elle and also *Harper's Bazaar* because of its crackly
paper and its luminous photos—it's very enjoyable.
A fashion series that made an impact on you?
In *Elle*, the extraordinary series on Jean-Paul
Goude for the Atlanta Olympics in 1996. It was
like a Hollywood-style super-production.
A cult fashion campaign? The Gucci campaign in
2004 by Guido Mocafico: snakes in extraordinary
colors were interlaced with the bags and shoes.
For or against photo touchups? For: when
you have to correct a few flaws; transcending
reality, ok. Against: when overdone to show
women disembodied, no longer anchored in
reality, and when this distances the reader
from the magazine; distorting reality, no!

———
Facing page: My advice
A phrase from Paul Valéry
"The void is always too much."
Envy is bad for your skin!

01
02
03
04
05
06
07
08
09
10
11
12
13
14
15
16
17
18
19
20
21

DAY

21

STAYING

Gorgeous forever

NEVER GIVE UP

FEED YOUR SOUL

"Never, never, never give up."

Winston Churchill

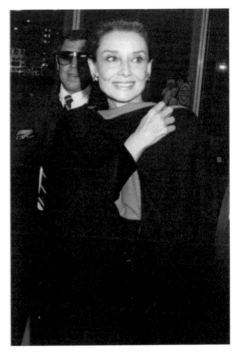

Audrey Hepburn.

N ever give up *what*, exactly? The desire to live, love, be interested, share, exchange views, and also, simply, the desire to please and be pleasing.

I have always loved older people, and aging has never scared me. Old age is a luxury that many people will never experience.

Benoîte Groult, a militant French feminist journalist and writer, tells a story of women and intergenerational relations in the beautiful book *La Touche étoile* ("the star touch," Grasset, 2004). She was eighty-six and described, with incredible finesse, the strange phenomenon she found herself faced with: the discrepancy between how others see her octogenarian body and the lively mind that is the same as it was when she was a young girl.

We now live longer than our ancestors, which is why it's important to keep believing and dreaming throughout our lives. Everything is always possible, and if we are at times faced with obstacles, we all have the inner resources to overcome them. By observing one hundred year old women, you'll notice many common denominators in them, like vitality,

the will to overcome, wonderful open-mindedness, and a beautiful smile.

Diet and a healthy lifestyle are fundamental, of course; we've talked about this throughout the book. Eating lightly, not compulsively, and keeping sugars and fats

21

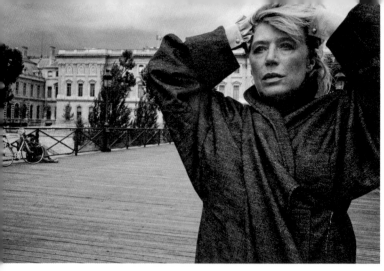

Facing page:
Lauren Hutton.

Left: Marianne Faithfull.

off your plate will help you live longer, just as it will if you avoid smoking and drinking. Exercising regularly is also a source of wellness. It's even more obvious as the years go by. Sports may not be a necessity when you are twenty, but they're essential as you age, so that you maintain a pretty figure, your joints in good shape, and your vital organs functioning properly. Exercise also procures peacefulness and relaxation for your mind and body. If you think it's too late or too hard, that's understandable, but get it into your head that it's just not true. Take Jane Fonda, for example, who at age forty-two managed to shape her body to look like a goddess.

Show commitment, and stop putting things off: set one goal per day and don't give it up, gradually it will become a habit, if not a need.

Before reviewing this advice for facing your mature years with panache, I wanted to give a twist to a preconceived idea that has caused much concern and even neurosis in some of us. As far back as I can remember, I was always terrified by the statement, which

you yourselves have most probably heard, that men age better than women. What an awful way of condemning women, and what a sad thing it is to imagine the future in such a negative way.

I firmly believe that there is nothing to it and that women absolutely do not age worse than men. If fresh features, supple skin, and a well-toned body do diminish as time wears on, you can still age with great style. There is nothing to stop you from attempting to keep your figure svelte. Coco Chanel is a good example of this. Also, there is nothing to stop you from staying nice and curvy. There is no "expiration date"; you can be beautiful and elegant at eighty. Don't listen to people who would have you think that, because of your advanced age, you should stop dressing extravagantly. Don't heed the advice of those who think it's better to cut your hair short when you're over fifty.

Let's put all these preconceived notions to rest and cheerfully look forward to becoming an inspiring, lively old lady with the spirit of a twenty year old.

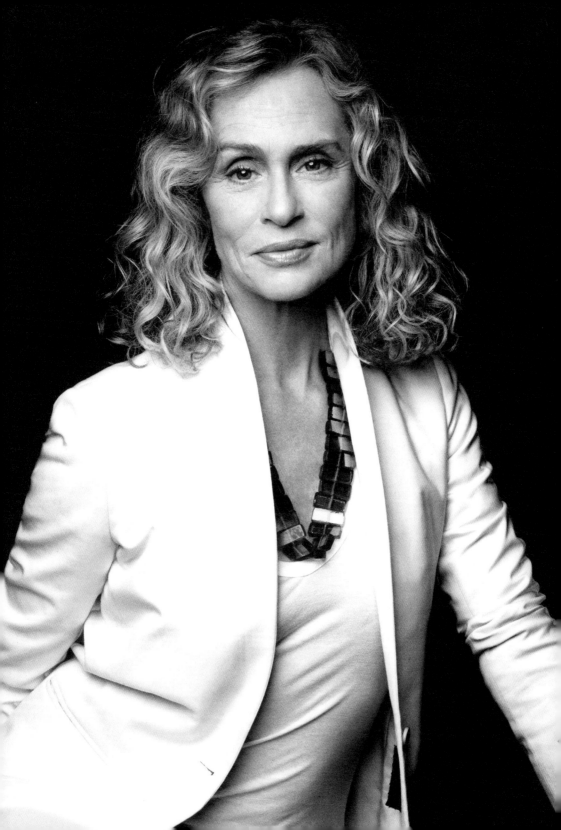

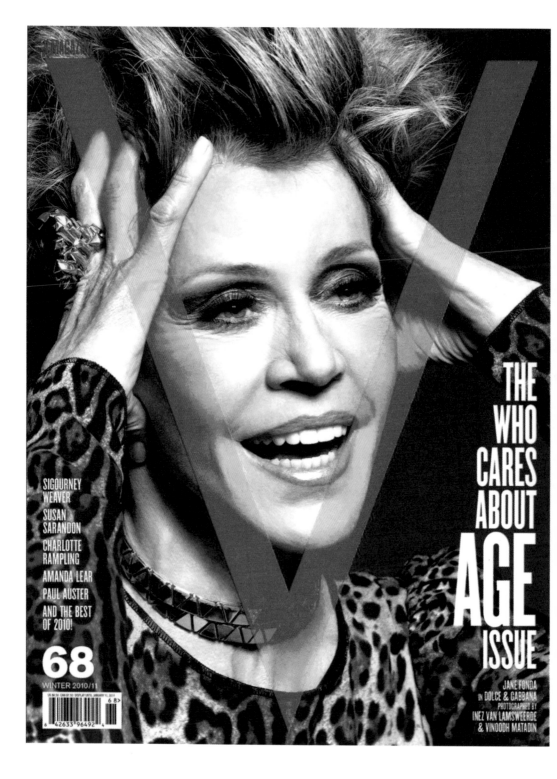

THE
WHO
CARES
ABOUT
AGE
ISSUE

SIGOURNEY
WEAVER

SUSAN
SARANDON

CHARLOTTE
RAMPLING

AMANDA LEAR

PAUL AUSTER

AND THE BEST
OF 2010!

68

WINTER 2010/11

JANE FONDA
IN DOLCE & GABBANA
PHOTOGRAPHED BY
INEZ VAN LAMSWEERDE
& VINOODH MATADIN

TO **LIVE WELL** AND **AGE WELL**

MAKE THE MOST OF IT

Starting now. Every moment is unique and won't come back.

HAVE PASSIONS

Get interested in the world. Be curious about everything. We can learn at any age: to play a musical instrument or to draw, for example. Be ready to explore things and the world.

TRAVEL

Exploring other cultures and landscapes is truly enriching.

BE POSITIVE

Have considerate relationships with people, be in tune with and in sync with yourself and others. Living well is to be at one with yourself, to do things with love.

BE RESPECTFUL

We are all responsible for the world around us, and if each of us pays attention to it, we will live better and longer. Respect yourself and others—these are social skills!

WORK HARD

To work is to do one or several jobs to earn your living, but not only. Whether it pays the bills or is the result of a passion—for a few lucky people—work is key in that it enables us to survive, to have access to a certain level of comfort. Do your work honestly and with love, and you'll doubly benefit from it. Be active. Get to work!

LOVE YOURSELF

To love yourself is to take time out for yourself; having just enough egoism to protect yourself from life's aggressions is one of the keys to existence.

LOVE OTHERS

Be good to your neighbors. This can seem like silly advice, but being altruistic and generous will make you better and make it easier for you to get along with others.

LOVE WITH A CAPITAL "L"

We are nothing without **Love**, that wonderful feeling that sweeps us up when we encounter it. Be in love, with the man in your life, your friends, your children! Every relationship is unique and precious, so give it your attention. Love makes us beautiful. It's the universal feeling that makes us all outdo ourselves. It's what drives us in life.

21

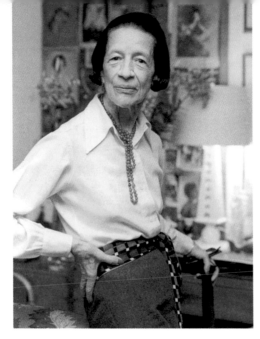

Diana Vreeland.

SMILE

Meet every day of your life with joy. Life is a gift, don't wait until it's too late to realize it. Throughout our lives, we come across moments of good luck, of hardship, we experience wonderful times and very difficult ones, and knowing how to keep a smile on your face in any circumstance is an attitude that will make you happier.

Don't whine over mere trifles. "Never explain, never complain," as Queen Victoria of England said to her son, the Prince of Wales, when he was ten. Positive, cheerful people attract others and the good things in life.

FIGHT BACK

Be indignant, not resigned. Rebel! Don't accept everything as inevitable. We are all masters of our destiny. It's up to you to change how things are going if you find them unsuitable. Be the heroine of your own life. Decide what is good for you and don't let others influence you. Knowing how to say no to others is, at times, a way of saying yes to yourself. Assert yourself, you are unique, so show yourself to advantage!

AND, FINALLY, DARE TO DREAM

Don't ever stop dreaming. My mother always said to me: "Life has more imagination than we do."

And that's right, we never know what the future holds for us, which is why you have to stay sharp and alert: "The best is yet to come!" Those adults who age well have all kept the soul of a child. They have that knack of being amazed by everything, and are ever at the ready to start all over again. Of believing in life like we used to believe in Santa Claus, having desire, being curious, laughing, loving, feeling free—that's the secret of eternal youth.

So for all these reasons and to live a long and wonderful life, NEVER GIVE UP! You have now completed the twenty-one day challenge. You have discovered your inner beauty and it shines forth. Whenever you feel you need a pick-me-up, and want to get gorgeous, you can start the challenge over again, to stay gorgeous forever.

DAY
21
MANTRAS

I put love and a positive attitude into:
....

I passionately love:
....

I'm grateful for:
....

I have a wonderful:
....

Today was this kind of day:
....

My superheroine name is:
....

I'm doing this with my life:
....

I LOVE MYSELF!

SHARE A PHOTO OF YOUR PERSONAL MANTRAS, THEN POST YOUR PHOTO
FROM DAY 1 WITH A PHOTO OF YOU TODAY. YOU'RE GORGEOUS !

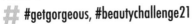 #getgorgeous, #beautychallenge21

This book is dedicated to Julien Bouyssou.

WITH THANKS TO:

Karuna Balloo, Olivia Blanckaert (Leonor Greyl), Harmony Boucher, Sara Brucker, Julie Chartier (Nice Work), Moïra Conrath, Amélie Cruchet (BPI), Gene Colon (La Roche Posay), Laura Di Maggio (La Prairie), Tamara Dolgieva (Lucien Pagès), Osana Ekue, Tiffanie Ereno (Serge Lutens), Fay, Caroline Fragner (Karl Lagerfeld), Muriel Frauciel (Yves Saint Laurent Beauty), Claude-Olivier Four, Julie Gaillard, Yona Grinbaum (Burberry), Jean-Albert Herman (Station-Service), Louise Hugault, Laure Hugonin (DM Media), Johanna (Les jardins de Nana), Alessandra Kapeluche, Pauline Klay, Jeremy Kouyaté, Tex Lacroix (Wrung), Selim Ladjimi (Sonia Rykiel), Marie Langlais (Guerlain), Marie-Laure Laporte (L'Oréal Luxe), Gaëlle Lassée, Léa Lauriol (Dior Parfums), Valerie Lecomte, Kimo & Tao Legia, Emily Le Moult (Caudalie), Tristan Lenormand, Patrick Lemire, Jean-François and Marie-Josée Loperena, Sophie Loperena, Pierre Macaigne (Lucien Pagès), Jeannine and Raymond Martin, Kate Mascaro, Carol Mason, Xavier Mauranne, Philippine Meites (Kiehl's), Catherine Miran, Christiane and Thierry Monnier, Max Monnier, Franck Mura, Ottavia Palomba, Françoise Pereira (Burberry), Françoise Pia, Lilo Quinel, Karyn Robert, Isabelle Safarian (Sisheido), Jonathan Sanchez, Vanessa Scoffier (Hôtel Henriette), Loïc Seailles (Puig), Johanne Sebag, Aymeline Valade, Gaëlle Vassilev (Caudalie), Jean-Luc Vatasso, Marie-Andrée and Roger Vatasso, Andréa Visini (Pressing).

AND SPECIAL THANKS TO THE EXPERTS:

Betty Autier, Yaz Bukey, Nathalie Cros-Coitton, Babeth Djian, Priscille d'Orgeval, Ana Girardot, Camille Hurel, Sylvia Jorif, Karolína Kurková, Noémie Lenoir, Karly Loyce, Margherita Missoni, Elisa Nalin, Soo Joo Park, Johanna Senyk, Daria Strokous, Victoire de Taillac, Mathilde Thomas, Aymeline Valade, and Kris Zero.

Creations by textile horticulturalist Karuna Balloo, featured on pp. 105 and 152, can be found on her website: www.karunaballoo.fr

The authors would also like to thank the locations that opened their doors to us for our photo shoots: pp. 58 (boxes), 151 (Maison Michel hat), 208, 214, and 215: Merci, 111 boulevard Beaumarchais, 75003 Paris, www.merci-merci.com/fr
pp. 209, 210, 212, and 213: Hôtel Henriette, 9 rue des Gobelins, 75013 Paris, www.hotelhenriette.com
pp. 105 and 211: Officine Universelle Buly 1803, 6 rue Bonaparte, 75006 Paris, www.buly1803.com

PHOTOGRAPHIC CREDITS

All photographs © Pascal Loperena and Christel Vatasso, with the exception of the following:
p. 9 Eileen Ford: © Nina Leen/Getty Images; p. 20 © Patrick Swirc; p. 28 Daniel Zuchnik/Getty Images; p. 40 © Pierre-Alban Hüe de Fontenay; p. 52 photo All rights reserved; p. 60 © Julia Champeau for Wanda Nylon; p. 72 © Caudalie; p. 84 © Leslie Kirchhoff; pp. 4–5 (bottom right) and 96 © Louise Carrasco; p. 109 © Franck Mura; p. 110 © Rasmus Skousen; p. 122 © Baldovino Barani; pp. 6 (bottom left) and 146 © Thomas Lavelle; p. 158 © Eric Guillemain; pp. 6 (top left), 7 (top right), 144, 152, 155, 163, 164, 167, 173–177, and 219 © Xavier Mauranne; p. 168 photo All rights reserved; p. 178 © Kirstin Sinclair/Getty Images; p. 186 © Tania et Vincent; p. 196 © Lucie Villemin; p. 204 © Alex Aristei; p. 216 © Fred Meylan; p. 223 © Yulia Reznikov/Shutterstock; p. 224 © Garance Doré; p. 230 © Sophie Steinberger; p. 233 © Time & Life Pictures/Getty Images; p. 234 Julian Broad/Getty Images; p. 235 © Fabrice Trombert/Getty Images; p. 238 © Bernard Gotfryd/Getty Images.

The inspiration tree reproduced on pp. 26–27 was created by Jérôme Colliard for Le Livre extraordinaire de -M- by Lisa Roze (Paris: Flammarion, 2011).

SOURCES

The definitions and quotations that appear on the chapter openers for days 2, 4, 11, 17, and 20 come from The Merriam-Webster Dictionary; La Mode pour les Nuls by Catherine Bézard (Paris: Éditions First-Gründ, 2012); Perfume: The Story of a Murderer by Patrick Süskind, trans. by John. E. Woods (London: Penguin, 2010); The Oxford Dictionary; and the Dictionnaire de l'Académie Française, respectively.